PHARMACOLOGY - RESEARCH, SAFETY TESTING AND REGULATION

DEXAMETHASONE

THERAPEUTIC USES, MECHANISM OF ACTION AND POTENTIAL SIDE EFFECTS

PHARMACOLOGY - RESEARCH, SAFETY TESTING AND REGULATION

Additional books in this series can be found on Nova's website under the Series tab.

Additional e-books in this series can be found on Nova's website under the e-book tab.

PHARMACOLOGY - RESEARCH, SAFETY TESTING AND REGULATION

DEXAMETHASONE

THERAPEUTIC USES, MECHANISM OF ACTION AND POTENTIAL SIDE EFFECTS

ALEXANDRE SAUVAGE

AND

MAXIME LEVY

EDITORS

NOVA BIOMEDICAL

New York

For permission to use material from this book please contact us:
Telephone 631-231-7269; Fax 631-231-8175
Web Site: http://www.novapublishers.com

Library of Congress Cataloging-in-Publication Data

ISBN: 978-1-62808-405-4
Library of Congress Control Number: 2013942945

Published by Nova Science Publishers, Inc. † New York

Contents

Preface

Dexamethasone is a potent, long-term acting synthetic glucocorticoid class of steroid drugs that have anti-inflammatory and immunosuppressant properties. The authors in this book discuss the therapeutic uses, mechanisms of action and potential side effects of dexamethasone. Topics include dexamethasone for the treatment of meconium aspiration syndrome (MAS); dexamethasone effects in hyperinfection syndrome due to strongyloidiasis; dexamethasone use in retinal disease and anti-tumor activities; perioperative uses of dexamethasone; comparison between cortisol and dexamethasone negative feed-back action in humans; the effect of dexamethasone on parathyroid hormone-related protein expression by oral cancer cells; and the effects of dexamethasone on the proliferation and differentiation of osteoblasts.

Chapter I – Dexamethasone is a potent, long-term acting synthetic glucocorticoid with wide use in the clinical practice. Dexamethasone, similarly to other glucocorticoids, exerts a lot of pharmacological properties useful in the treatment of inflammation, lung edema, and pulmonary vasoconstriction in the meconium-injured lungs. Whereas an inflammation plays a significant role in the pathogenesis of neonatal meconium aspiration syndrome (MAS), dexamethasone has been used also in this indication. Nevertheless, despite growing information on positive effects of dexamethasone administration in MAS, many questions have not been answered yet, e.g. on possible adverse effects of the treatment. To consider objectively the positives and negatives of dexamethasone use in MAS, this chapter reviews the pathomechanims of MAS, mechanisms of action of glucocorticoids and dexamethasone, and experience with delivery of dexamethasone in the experimental models and in the newborns with MAS including the side effects of the treatment. Chapter II – Background: Dexamethasone is a synthetic corticosteroid with anti-inflammatory effects that is widely used to treat autoimmune and other chronic inflammatory diseases. Prolonged treatment with dexamethasone can result in the development of hyperinfection syndrome in strongyloidiasis through several different mechanisms. This complication can be relevant in areas where *Strongyloides* species are endemic, rendering hyperinfection syndrome an important global health problem. Material and Methods: Rats inoculated with 9×10^3 *Strongyloides venezuelensis* larvae and treated with dexamethasone were sacrificed on days 1, 3, 5, 7, 14 and 21. The lungs, spleen, kidney, heart, liver, and brain were harvested, minced and incubated, so that migrating larvae could be collected and counted under a light microscope. Eosinophils and mononuclear cells were quantified from blood samples, BALF (bronchoalveolar lavage fluid) and PCF (peritoneal cavity fluid). Interleukin levels were evaluated using an ELISA assay. Corticosterone and ecdysteroid were measured in parasite cultures. Glucocorticoid receptor protein levels were assessed in parasite extracts by Western immunoblot analysis. Results: Dexamethasone-treated rats carried increased parasite burdens and had enhanced female worm fertility, which induced steroid-hormone overproduction by the parasites, likely via an increase in the synthesis of corticosterone and ecdysone-like hormones. Dexamethasone also reduced eosinophil and mononuclear cell numbers and inhibited interleukins such as IL-1β and IL-4, culminating with the dissemination of larvae to other organs indicating a progression toward hyperinfection and death. Conclusion: Dexamethasone decreases the Th2-type immune response to parasitic infection, ultimately leading to septic shock and the dissemination of larvae to other organs. Furthermore, dexamethasone may play a direct role in promoting worm proliferation. Further experimental studies are essential to elucidate the parasite's behavior and the role of the immune system in strongyloidiasis, particularly in patients using dexamethasone to treat hyperinfection syndrome. These studies contribute to the understanding of the molecular basis of infection and help to prevent hyperinfection syndrome in strongyloidiasis, which has a high mortality rate.

Chapter III – Steroids, having both anti-inflammatory and anti-angiogenic properties, are a useful therapeutic option in the treatment of retinal disease. Intravitreal steroids can be used in the treatment of various retinal conditions including diabetic and vasculo-occlusive macular edema, exudative macular degeneration, pseudophakic cystoid macular edema, and posterior uveitis. Although there are well known serious potential complications with intravitreal steroids, including glaucoma and endophthalmitis, recent studies have shown that intravitreal steroids may be used as a safe alternative to the practice of laser therapy for the treatment of macular edema secondary to diabetes or vein occlusions. Although there are several steroid formulations that may be used, this article focuses on the use of intravitreal dexamethasone. Dexamethasone is a potent anti-inflammatory agent that inhibits multiple inflammatory cytokines. Despite its established therapeutic benefit, side effects such as cataract formation and ocular hypertension/glaucoma raise concerns. Therefore, understanding the molecular and genetic effects of intraocular steroid treatments is of utmost importance and of clinical relevance. Our *in vivo* studies have elucidated several genes and pathways that are potentially altering the neuroprotective and/or neurodegenerative balance between glial and retinal ganglion cells during intravitreal steroid treatment, such as semaphorin signaling, a member of the neuronal axonal guidance signaling system. Furthermore, our more recent data results suggests that dexamethasone affects the balance of Th1, Th2 and Th17 cytokine production, which influences many pathological processes and plays both causative and protective roles in retinal disease.

Chapter IV – It is well known that dexamethasone (DEX) and other glucocorticoids are of great value in the treatment of various pathologic conditions, including inflammatory disorders and autoimmune diseases. In patients with solid tumors, a glucocorticoid is often prescribed, for instance, to reduce side effects of chemotherapeutic agents and to improve cachectic conditions. DEX, given alone or in combination with other drugs, has also been clinically used as a direct chemotherapeutic agent, primarily in hematological malignancies such as multiple myeloma and acute lymphocytic leukemia. In contrast, cytotoxic activities of DEX on solid tumors remain poorly characterized. Nonetheless, recent experimental data have suggested its direct effects on cell growth of solid tumors, such as prostate and bladder carcinomas. Indeed, in patients with castration-resistant prostate cancer, DEX treatment with or without docetaxel has been shown to prolong their survival. This chapter reviews clinical and molecular evidence supporting anti-tumor properties of DEX.

Chapter V – Dexamethasone is a synthetic glucocorticoid with an established role as an anti-inflammatory, immunosuppressant, and agent to prevent post operative nausea and vomiting. More recent evidence has demonstrated a potential role for dexamethasone in postoperative pain management, both as a systemic analgesic and adjuvant to local anesthetics for perineural use. Dexamethasone binds to glucocorticoid receptors in the cytoplasm, dimerizes and then translocates into the nucleus. In the nucleus, it binds to specific DNA sequences to regulate gene transcription of agents involved in the function of inflammatory response mediators, such as cytokines, arachidonic acid and endothelial leukocyte adhesion molecules. Compared to other glucocorticoids, dexamethasone has the strongest anti-inflammatory effect with 30 times the potency of hydrocortisone. Dexamethasone has also shown to be useful in the treatment of nausea and vomiting by altering phospholipase A2 synthesis thus suppressing prostaglandin production. It is also believed that the reduction of circulating inflammatory mediators that can stimulate the chemoreceptor trigger zone in the brain may also contribute to this effect. Moreover, a single preoperative dose of dexamethasone has shown to be an effective adjunct to reduce postoperative pain and opioid consumption after surgery. Lower pain scores might be explained by its inhibitory effect on prostaglandin production. Additionally, with the suppression of inflammatory mediators, activation of peripheral pain receptors is limited. In the same way, the use of dexamethasone with local anesthetics has been demonstrated to significantly prolong the analgesic effect of nerve blocks either by inducing vasoconstriction and thus reducing local anesthetic absorption or by increasing the activity of inhibitory potassium channels on nociceptive c-fibers, thus decreasing their activity. Although the benefits of glucocorticoids are well known, prolonged use or high doses have significant adverse effects. Dexamethasone, as all glucocorticoids, increases levels of glucose in the blood potentially leading to glucocorticoid-induced diabetes. Extended use also can cause hypertension via renal sodium retention and potentiation of vasopressor responses to angiotensin II and catecholamines. Additionally, it reduces the proliferation of chondrocytes inducing the apoptosis of these cells thus slowing down the growth rate in children. In adults, osteoporosis and increased risk of fractures are side effects related with prolonged use. The repair and healing of aseptic wounds is also inhibited or delayed by dexamethasone, which not only blocks cytokine signaling but also inhibits the synthesis of collagen and other important factors in wound repair. Moreover, there is evidence of suppression of the hypothalamic-pituitary axis and development of glucocorticoid resistance after prolonged use of this glucocorticoid. Therefore, even though the utility of dexamethasone as an anti-inflammatory, immunosuppressive, and analgesic agent is evident, the hazards of its use must also be appreciated. This review will summarize the evidence for the use of dexamethasone in anesthesiology and acute pain management. Molecular mechanisms (where known) will be discussed. Potential hazards and areas of uncertainty will be explored, as will future avenues of research.

Chapter VI – Glucocorticoids (GCs) inhibit HPA axis through different mechanisms and target sites mediated by two receptor types (glucocorticoid receptor, GR, and mineralcorticoid receptor, MR). Within the brain, GRs are mostly distributed in the hypothalamus and in the pituitary, and bind both natural and synthetic GCs; MRs are mainly located in the limbic structures where show high affinity for GCs. HPA response to GCs feedback is usually tested by dexamethasone, a synthetic GC that poorly penetrates BBB and preferentially activates pituitaric GRs. Differently from dexamethasone, cortisol could better evaluate the GC feedback action by acting also at supra-pituitary level. We studied the effects of different doses of hydrocortisone (HC, 15, 30 or 60 μg/kg/h, infused for 150 min) or dexamethasone (DEX, 0.4, 0.8 or 1.6 μg/kg/h, infused for 150 min) on ACTH and cortisol levels in 6 normal subjects (NS, age 25±2.1 yr, BMI 23.0±1.2 kg/m^2). The effects of HC and DEX were compared with those of placebo. Blood samples were taken every 15 min for 240 min. During placebo, ACTH and cortisol levels showed progressive decrease (baseline vs nadir, mean±SEM: 17.6±1.6 vs 13.4±0.7 pg/ml and 157.6±25.6 vs 71.7±10.6 μg/l, $p<0.05$). The dose of 15 μg/kg/h HC mantained constant cortisol but did not modify ACTH levels at any time. The doses of 30 and 60 μg/kg/h HC induced dose-dependent cortisol increases (peaks, 30 μg/kg/h: 170.5±14.8 μg/l, $p<0.05$; 60 μg/kg/h: 203.2±26.6 μg/l, $p<0.05$) associated to dose-dependent ACTH decrease (nadir, 30 μg/kg/h: 8.1±0.9 pg/ml, $p<0.05$; 60 μg/kg/h: 7.9±0.7 pg/ml, $p<0.05$). DEX at doses of 0.4, 0.8 and 1.6 μg/kg/h did not modify cortisol levels at any time. Only 1.6 μg/kg/h DEX induced an ACTH decrease ($p<0.05$) more pronounced than that after placebo (8.0±3.1 pg/ml) while neither 0.4 nor 0.8 μg/kg/h affected ACTH levels at any time. In conclusion, taking into account the potency at the GR level, doses of dexamethasone relatively higher than hydrocortisone are needed to inhibit ACTH secretion in humans. These findings are likely to reflect different sites where natural and synthetic GCs exert their feedback action, i.e. mainly the CNS for cortisol and the pituitary for dexamethasone. It is suggested that the HPA sensitivity to the feedback action of GCs in various pathophysiological conditions would better be evaluated by using natural GCs.

Chapter VII – Parathyroid hormone-related protein (PTHrP) is known to act as a major causative factor for humoral hypercalcemia of malignancy (HHM). Production of PTHrP is up-regulated in certain malignancies and elevated PTHrP expression has been correlated with advanced disease and a poor prognosis. Therefore, down-regulation of PTHrP production in cancer cells is important to provide an approach for prevention of HHM. But there is little effective treatment for controlling the increased production of PTHrP in cancer cells. Glucocorticoids (including dexamethasone) exhibit diverse biological activities, such as anti-inflammatory and immunosuppressive effects on various cells and tissues. There is also considerable interest in application of glucocorticoids to cancer treatment. In the latest research using HSC-3, a human oral squamous carcinoma cell line, it was demonstrated that dexamethasone suppresses PTHrP mRNA expression and PTHrP production in a dose-dependent manner. Furthermore, dexamethasone was shown to act through binding to functional glucocorticoid receptors and down-regulate PTHrP gene expression via a transcriptional mechanism in HSC-3 cells. Application of dexamethasone may become a new strategy for preventing PTHrP-induced HHM .

Chapter VIII – Dexamethasone is reported to be a potent synthetic member of the glucocorticoid class of steroid drugs. It acts as an anti-inflammatory and immunosuppressant. Glucocorticoid is reported to induce osteoporosis. On the other hand, several studies have demonstrated that dexamethasone increased the bone formation capacity of osteoprogenitor cells *in vitro*. The effects of dexamethasone on the proliferation, activity, and cytokine secretion of normal human bone marrow stromal cells were tested, and alkaline phosphatase activity was markedly stimulated with the addition of dexamethasone. The diverse and complex effects on bone metabolism are still not completely understood. In this paper, an extensive review of the role of dexamethasone regarding osteoblast and bone marrow stromal cells will be performed using *in vitro* and *in vivo* studies. Clinical implications of dexamethasone will be also conducted.

In: Dexamethasone
Editors: A. Sauvage and M. Levy

ISBN: 978-1-62808-405-4

Chapter I

Dexamethasone in the Treatment of Meconium Aspiration Syndrome: Benefits versus Side Effects

Daniela Mokra[1,*], Juraj Mokry[2] and Ingrid Tonhajzerova[1]

[1]Department of Physiology, Jessenius Faculty of Medicine, Comenius University, Martin, Slovakia

[2]Department of Pharmacology, Jessenius Faculty of Medicine, Comenius University, Martin, Slovakia

Abstract

Dexamethasone is a potent, long-term acting synthetic glucocorticoid with wide use in the clinical practice. Dexamethasone, similarly to other glucocorticoids, exerts a lot of pharmacological properties useful in the treatment of inflammation, lung edema, and pulmonary vasoconstriction in the meconium-injured lungs. Whereas an inflammation plays a

[*] Corresponding author: Daniela Mokra, MD, PhD, Department of Physiology, Jessenius Faculty of Medicine, Comenius University, Mala Hora 4, 03601 Martin, Slovakia, EU, Phone: +421 43 2633454, E-mail: mokra@jfmed.uniba.sk.

significant role in the pathogenesis of neonatal meconium aspiration syndrome (MAS), dexamethasone has been used also in this indication. Nevertheless, despite growing information on positive effects of dexamethasone administration in MAS, many questions have not been answered yet, e.g. on possible adverse effects of the treatment. To consider objectively the positives and negatives of dexamethasone use in MAS, this chapter reviews the pathomechanims of MAS, mechanisms of action of glucocorticoids and dexamethasone, and experience with delivery of dexamethasone in the experimental models and in the newborns with MAS including the side effects of the treatment.

Keywords: Dexamethasone, glucocorticoids, meconium aspiration syndrome, animal model, newborn

List of Abbreviations

AP-1	protein activator-1
ATP	adenosine triphosphate
BAL	bronchoalveolar lavage
cGR	cytoplasmic glucocorticoid receptor
COPD	chronic obstructive pulmonary disease
COX	cyclooxygenase
DNA	deoxyribonucleic acid
ENaC	epithelial Na^+ channels
ET-1	endothelin 1
FiO_2	fraction of inspired oxygen
GC	glucocorticoid
GCs	glucocorticoids
GM-CSF	granulocyte-monocyte colony stimulating factor
GR	glucocorticoid receptor
GRE	glucocorticoid responsive element
HDAC	histone deacetylase
HPA	hypothalamic – pituitary - adrenal
11β-HSD	11β-hydroxysteroid dehydrogenase
HSP90	heat shock protein 90
ICAM	intercellular adhesion molecule
IL	interleukin
iNOS	inducible nitric oxide synthase
JNK	c-Jun terminal kinase

LPS	lipopolysaccharide
LT	leukotriene
MAPK	mitogen activated protein kinase
MAS	meconium aspiration syndrome
mGR	membrane-bound glucocorticoid receptor
MIP	macrophage inflammatory protein
MR	mineralocorticoid receptor
mRNA	mitochondrial ribonucleic acid
NF-κB	nuclear factor κB
NO	nitric oxide
PAF	platelet activating factor
$PaCO_2$	partial pressure of carbon dioxide in the arterial blood
PaO_2	partial pressure of oxygen in the arterial blood
PG	prostaglandin
PLA_2	phospholipase A_2
RONS	reactive oxygen and nitrogen species
SEGRA	selective glucocorticoid receptor agonists
SLPI	secretory leukocyte proteinase inhibitor
SP-B	specific surfactant protein B
TAS	total antioxidant status
TBARS	thiobarbituric acid-reactive substances
TGFβ	transforming growth factor β
TNFα	tumor necrosis factor α
TXA_2	thromboxane A_2

Introduction

Meconium Aspiration Syndrome (MAS)

Meconium passage and meconium aspiration

Meconium aspiration syndrome (MAS) is a serious respiratory disorder occuring particularly in the term and post-term newborns. Meconium, the first faeces of the newborn, is a dark-green, viscous mixture of amniotic fluid, desquamated cells, lanugo, vernix caseosa, mucus, and gastrointestinal secretes. Biochemically, meconium contains mucopolysaccharides, bile acids, bile salts, bilirubin, cholesterol, free fatty acids, gastrointestinal enzymes including pancreatic phospholipase A_2, tri-, di- and monoglycerides [Co and

Vidyasagar 1990]. In addition, meconium is a source of various pro-inflammatory substances, such as interleukins (IL) -1, -6, and -8, and tumor necrosis factor (TNF)α (de Beaufort et al. 2003). Meconium is produced in the fetal intestine since 10th-12th gestational week, however, spontaneous evacuation of meconium into the amniotic fluid is rare because of lack of strong peristalsis, presence of a tonic contraction of anal sphincter, and presence of terminal plug of highly viscous meconium (Fuloria and Wiswell 1999). Occurence of meconium in the amniotic fluid increases with increasing gestational age and may be caused by several factors. First, meconium appearance in the amniotic fluid is historically considered to be an indicator of the fetal maturation (Katz and Bowes 1992). Passage of meconium into the amniotic fluid may be accelerated by neuronal myelinization, maturation of the parasympathetic part of the autonomic nervous system and/or increasing concentration of motiline, a hormone speeding up the peristalsis and defecation (Klingner and Kruse 1999). Furthermore, meconium may be released also due to vagal stimulation following a compression of the fetal head or umbilical cord, finally leading to facilitated gastrointestinal motility (Wiswell and Bent 1993). Nevertheless, passage of meconium is frequently associated with a fetal distress. Hypoxia causes centralization of the blood flow through the vitally important organs and vasoconstriction in less important ones, including intestines. Intestinal ischemia transiently stimulates the peristalsis and relaxation of anal sphincter (Co and Vidyasagar 1990). In addition, asphyxia in fetus potentiates the respiratory movements, and thereby increases the risk of aspiration of meconium-stained amniotic fluid (Blackburn and Loper 1992). However, chronic intrauterine hypoxia causes severe ischemic changes on placenta and excessive muscularization of pulmonary arteries and intralobular arterioles, leading to pulmonary hypertension immediately after the labour (Thureen et al. 1997). In such cases, presence of meconium in the amniotic fluid and its aspiration is more an indicator of chronic distress than the primary cause of the disorder (Wiswell and Bent 1993). Regardless the primary cause, aspiration of meconium may lead to serious short-term and long-term adverse effects. Although meconium-stained amniotic fluid appears in 10-15 % of all newborns, MAS develops in about 3-5 % of them. The question, why some newborns born through the meconium-stained amniotic fluid develop MAS and other not, is still unanswered. Higher risk of MAS development was described in black ethnic, higher gestational age and birth weight, male gender, or in fetal compromise. Clinical signs of the disorder vary in severity from mild tachypnoe to severe respiratory failure with hypoxemia and hypercarbia, associated with pulmonary hypertension

(Dargaville et al. 2006, van Ierland and de Beaufort 2009). In addition to acute effects, MAS may cause also serious long-term consequences on the respiratory system, whereas abnormal bronchial reactivity, wheezing and other respiratory pathology were found in a significant portion of infants who had overcome MAS in the neonatal period (Vázquez Nava et al. 2006).

Pathomechanisms of MAS

Pathophysiology of MAS is complex with multiple interactions between the individual pathomechanisms: mechanical obstruction of the airways, dysfunction of pulmonary surfactant, meconium-induced inflammation, lung edema, and pulmonary vasoconstriction often leading to persistent pulmonary hypertension. Additionally, process of meconium-induced lung injury interferes with perinatal changes of the fluid-filled lungs to air-filled organ, required for an adequate gas exchange (van Ierland and de Beaufort 2009).

In an acute phase of the disease, aspirated meconium obstructs the airways. Complete airway obstruction by thick meconium results in an alveolar atelectasis behind the plug. Partial airway obstruction causes a ball-valve effect, with air-trapping and risk of air leak into the interstitium (Tyler et al. 1978, Tran et al. 1980). Areas of the lungs which do not participate in ventilation become hypoxic. Perfusion of non-ventilated alveoli increases right-to-left pulmonary shunts and potentiates hypoxemia, and in severe cases also the return to a fetal type of circulation (Bacsik 1977, Co and Vidyasagar 1990).

When reaches the alveoli, meconium triggers inflammation (Wu et al. 1999). As a potent chemoattractant for neutrophils (Yamada et al. 2000), meconium increases number of neutrophils in the lungs within several hours after the aspiration, what is linked with their decrease in the blood (Soukka et al. 1997, Mokry et al. 2006). Meconium induces lung inflammation directly or indirectly through the stimulation of oxidative burst and production of pro-inflammatory cytokines (IL-1β, IL-6, IL-8, and TNFα) in the lungs (Soukka et al. 2002, Craig et al. 2005, Zagariya et al. 2004). Released cytokines from activated macrophages enhance adhesion of neutrophils on the endothelium and formation the microemboli in the capillary bed, participating in the onset of pulmonary hypertension. This process is facilitated by a complement, which activation has been proven also in MAS (Castellheim et al. 2005). Activated leukocytes, platelets, epithelial and endothelial cells produce a wide spectrum of substances, such as TNFα, IL, leukotrienes (LT), prostaglandins (PG), platelet activating factor (PAF), proteolytic enzymes, reactive oxygen and nitrogen species (RONS) etc., deteriorating the lung parenchyma and surfactant. Inflammatory cytokines induce expression of angiotensin II, one of factors responsible for apoptosis of the lung cells after its binding to angiotensin II type 1 receptors (Vidyasagar and Zagariya 2008). Meconium contains high concentrations of phospholipase A_2 (PLA_2), which directly or via arachidonic acid metabolism increases the production of lipid mediators and participates in the surfactant dysfunction (Schrama et al. 2001) and apoptosis of epithelial cells (Holopainen et al. 1999). Nevertheless, intensive apoptosis of the lung cells may be caused by nitric oxide, angiotensin II, ROS and other factors, as well (Vidyasagar et al. 2005, Zagariya et al. 2005, Zagariya et al. 2006, Vidyasagar and Zagariya 2008). Meconium enhances expression of inducible cyclooxygenase-2 (COX-2) and inducible nitric oxide synthase (iNOS) in the macrophages, epithelial and endothelial cells (Uotila and Kääpä 1999, Li et al. 2001, Kytola et al. 2003, Fontanilla et al. 2008). Furthermore, a release of bronchoactive substances, such as LT and PAF, probably participates in an airway hyperreactivity to bronchoconstrictors (Khan et al. 2002a, Mokry et al. 2006).

In addition, components of meconium (cholesterol, free fatty acids, bile acids, lysophospholipids, bilirubin etc.) interfere with a surfactant ability to reduce the surface tension at air:liquid interphase during compression of the surface and fluidize the surfactant film (Diemel et al. 2002, Zuo et al. 2008). For example, bile acids penetrate through the lamelar structures and surfactant monolayer and alleviate a leak of cholesterol into the surfactant complexes and injure their function (Lopez-Rodriguez et al. 2011). High concentrations of bile acids increase the production and activation of phospholipase A_2 in the lungs. PLA_2 may then directly or indirectly through its products, such as lysophosholipids, affect the surfactant metabolism and damage the cell membranes (De Luca et al. 2011).

Dysfunction of surfactant is potentiated by plasma proteins leaking through injured alveolocapillary membrane. Plasma proteins may deteriorate surfactant function via several mechanisms. Albumin, fibrinogen and hemoglobin inhibit surfactant function through competitive adsorption with surfactant phospholipids at an air:liquid interphase (Holm et al. 1999). Furthermore, albumin interacts with double-layer of phospholipids and thereby interrupts their distribution in the structures of surfactant (Larsson et al. 2006), and C-reactive protein fluidizes the surfactant film (Sáenz et al. 2010).

Pulmonary surfactant may be inactivated also by action of proteolytic enzymes and RONS released from activated cells during the inflammation. In the previous studies, TNFα and IL-1 inhibited expression of surfactant proteins (Hallman et al., 2001), and RONS damaged both the surfactant proteins and phospholipids (Rodríguez-Capote et al. 2006). Structure and function of surfactant may be enzymatically degraded also by proteolytic enzymes including phospholipase A_2 (De Luca et al. 2011).

Meconium aspiration is often associated with pulmonary vasoconstriction from hypoxia and/or from direct vasoconstriction effect of meconium and substances released in inflammation. Presence of meconium in the fetal amniotic fluid may cause ischemic changes of the lungs, umbilical cord, and placenta (Burgess and Hutchins 1996). Postnatal meconium instillation elevates the pulmonary artery pressure and vascular resistance in a concentration-dependent manner (Holopainen et al. 1998), what is linked with higher levels of thromboxane A_2 (TXA_2), LT, PG, and endothelin-1 (ET-1) (Soukka et al. 1998b, Kuo and Chen 1999, Wu et al. 1999).

Subsequently, as a result of the complex influence of surfactant dysfunction, inflammation, and oxidation injury, leak of proteinaceous fluid and cells into the alveolar spaces through the alveolocapillary membrane further deteriorate the lung functions.

Treatment Options in MAS

Because of complex pathophysiology of the disease, treatment of MAS is still problematic. In the last decades, many adjunctive or alternative approaches have been tested in MAS (Mokra and Mokry 2010). Since some of them have been well established, e.g. ventilatory support, different modes of artificial ventilation including high-frequency ventilation (Tingay et al. 2007, Goldsmith 2008, Dargaville 2012a) and liquid ventilation (Jeng et al. 2006, Avoine et al. 2011), administration of exogenous surfactant as a bolus or lung lavage (Dargaville and Mills 2005, Dargaville 2012b), or inhaled nitric oxide (Steinhorn 2008, Dargaville 2012a), therapeutic potential of others, e.g. anti-inflammatory drugs and vasodilators is still under research (Asad and Bhat 2008, Geiger et al. 2008, Kääpä 2009, Silvera et al. 2011, Rey-Santano et al. 2012).

Glucocorticoids in the Treatment of MAS

Among all anti-inflammatory drugs already tested in MAS, glucocorticoids (GCs) have an exceptional position, as they may affect several pathomechanisms of MAS at once. GCs reduce penetration of neutrophils into the lungs decreasing their adherence to the endothelium and suppress their activation. GCs also diminish numbers of circulating mononuclears, eosinophils, and basophils and decrease synthesis of cytokines by macrophages, eosinophils, and T-lymphocytes. In addition, GCs stabilize lysosomes, inhibit a release of lysosomal enzymes, and influence chemotaxia and other functions of neutrophils. Stabilizing cell membranes and decreasing production of pro-inflammatory and vasoactive substances GCs reduce microvascular permeability. Moreover, modulating the pulmonary vasomotoric tone GCs alleviate pulmonary vasoconstriction and inhibit fibrogenesis (Jantz and Sahn, 1999, Fernandes et al. 2005, Czock et al. 2005). Whereas GCs affect also the cardiovascular system and metabolism in stressful situations, adaptive responses such as keeping blood pressure and recruiting glucose to supply energy might be considered as additional advantages of GCs administration in the newborns suffering from MAS.

In the further subsections, general mechanisms of action of GCs, pharmacological properties of dexamethasone, a glucocorticoid preparation most frequently used in MAS, as well as desirable and side effects of dexamethasone treatment in MAS are reviewed.

Pharmacological Properties of GCs, Pharmacokinetics and Pharmacodynamics of GCs

Endogenous GCs play a fundamental role in the response to stress including trauma, sepsis, starvation, tissue ischemia, and to mental stress. Such stimulation activates hypothalamic-pituitary-adrenal (HPA) axis and results in release of cortisol. Cortisol mediates its effects via activation of intracellular glucocorticoid (GR) receptors, which are expressed ubiquitously (Walker 2007a). In addition, cortisol interacts with mineralocorticoid (MR) receptors, which are expressed only in selected tissues and at lower levels. In some tissues (distal nephron, vascular endothelium etc.), MRs bind exclusively aldosterone, as cortisol is excluded by local pre-receptor inactivation by 11β-hydroxysteroid dehydrogenase type 2 (HSD2) to inert cortisone. Contrary in myocardium, vascular smooth muscle or adipose tissue, MRs are occupied by cortisol in competition with much lower prevailing concentrations of aldosterone and active cortisol regenerates from inactive cortisone under the influence of 11β-HSD1 amplifying GR activation (Tomlinson et al. 2004, Walker 2007a). Thus, 11β-HSD1 acts as a reductase converting inactive cortisone to active cortisol in the cells. The mentioned intracellular MRs and GCs receptors act as transcription factors on approximately one third of genes, as the pattern of response in individual cell types depends on the complexity of interactions with heterodimers, co-activators and co-repressors, and epigenetic factors including chromatin organisation (Walker 2007a).

Pharmacokinetic properties of GCs depend on their physico-chemical characteristics (Mager and Jusko 2002). GCs preparation generally includes hydrophilic phosphate and succinate ester of GCs, which is converted within 5-30 min to its active form (Czock et al. 2005).

Glucocorticoids are well absorbed after oral administration and have a bioavailability of 60-100% (61-86% for orally administered dexamethasone), however, intravenous administration increases it to >90%. While the pharmacokinetics of hydrocortisone (cortisol) and prednisolone are non-linear, that of dexamethasone after intravenous administration is linear (Rohdewald et al. 1987). This special feature is caused by the fact that dexamethasone has no affinity for transcortin (corticosteroid binding glubulin) and binds only to albumin (75 % of circulating dexamethasone is bond to albumin) (Cummings et al. 1990). Contrary, hydrocortisone and prednisolone bind to both transcortin and albumin. Protein binding is biologically relevant, because only free drug is able to reach the biological effect, i.e. to reach the active site and to interact with a receptor involved in its action. Thus, pharmacokinetic properties should be considered in expecting the pharmacodynamic properties. Despite relatively low impact of alteration in protein binding on GCs action, in some cases low plasma albumin concentration can lead to enhanced drug action and to increased occurence of adverse effects (Lewis et al., 1971).

The metabolism and excretion of GCs is a two-step process, i.e. after adding the oxygen and hydrogen atoms conjugation (glucuronidation or sulphation) occures. Final hydrophilic inactive metabolites are excreted by kidneys. Only 1-20 % of unchanged GCs are excreted (Czock et al. 2005). The comparison of some pharmacokinetic parameters after intravenous administration of the most important glucocorticoids is shown in *Table 1*.

Table 1. Pharmacokinetic parameters of GCs after intravenous systemic administration (C_{max} – peak plasma concentration of GC, $T_{1/2}$ – terminal half-life, V_d – volume of distribution, Cl – total clearance, PB – plasma binding, f_{ren} – renally excreted fraction of unchanged drug; *C_{max} was normalised to a GC dose of 1 mg; &volume and clearance parameters are normalised to 70 kg b.w.). Adapted from (Czock et al., 2005)

	C_{max}* (μg/L)	$T_{1/2}$ (h)	Vd& (L)	Cl& (L/h)	PB (%)	f_{ren} (%)
Hydrocortisone	15.3±2.9	2.0±0.3	27±7	18±4	92±2	
Prednisolone phosphate	88.3±24.0	3.0±0.4	45±5	9±2	73±4	18.0±6.6
Methyloprednisolone succinate	8.3±3.3	2.4±0.6	75±16	24±7	78±2	9.2±0.7
Dexamethasone sodium phosphate	10.5±2.8	4.6±1.2	65.7±17.3	12±4	75±4	

As mentioned above, most of GCs are able, in some extent, to stimulate MR receptors. This effect can be pronounced when the capacity of 11β-HSD2, an enzyme involved in the control of availability of GCs for binding to GR and MR receptors, is exceeded. While 11β-HSD1 acting predominantly as a reductase converts inactive cortisone to active cortisol, 11β-HSD2 converts by oxidation cortisol to cortisone, thus preventing action of cortisol on MR receptors (Diederich et al., 2002). From this point of view, bolus administration of higher doses of GCs exceeding the capacity of 11β-HSD2 and saturating MR receptors may enhance their mineralocorticoid effect. On the other hand, a low glucocorticoid dose leading to intracellular concentrations just above the protective capacity of this enzyme would be expected to have reduced mineralocorticoid effects (Czock et al., 2005). Comparison of pharmacological effectiveness of major GCs is presented in *Table 2*.

As the pharmacokinetics of GCs is not very specific, several drug-drug interactions and diseases play an important role in the final effect of GCs. Co-administration of enzyme inducers (e.g. barbiturates, carbamazepine, phenytoin, rifampicin) leads to increase of clearance and decrease of half-life of prednisolone and methylprednisolone. For dexamethasone, co-administration of cytochrome P450 3A4 inhibitors (ketoconazole, itraconazole, clarithromycine) should be considered; itraconazole decreased the clearance to 30 % and increased three-times the half-life of dexamethasone. Comparable changes were observed with methylprednisolone administration, but not with prednisolone. Nevertheless, short-term administration of macrolides does not require a dose reduction of GCs. Similarly, smoking does not affect the pharmacokinetics of dexamethasone (Rose et al., 1981).

Table 2. Basic characteristics of commonly used natural and synthetic corticosteroids (Katzung et al., 2012)

Agent	Activity			Equivalent Oral Dose (mg)	Forms Available
	Anti-inflammatory	Topical	Salt-retaining		
Short- to medium-acting GCs					
Hydrocortisone (cortisol)	1	1	1	20	p.o., inj., top.
Cortisone	0.8	0	0.8	25	p.o.
Prednisone	4	0	0.3	5	p.o., inj.
Prednisolone	5	4	0.3	5	p.o., inj.
Methylprednisolone	5	5	0	4	p.o., inj.
Meprednisone	5	-	0	4	p.o., inj.
Intermediate-acting GCs					
Triamcinolone	5	5	0	4	p.o., inj., top.
Paramethasone	10	-	0	2	p.o., inj.
Fluprednisolone	15	7	0	1.5	p.o.
Long-acting GCs					
Betamethasone	25-40	10	0	0.6	p.o., inj., top.
Dexamethasone	30	10	0	0.75	p.o., inj., top.
Mineralocorticoids					
Fludrocortisone	10	0	250	2	p.o.
Desoxycorticosterone acetate	0	0	20	-	p.o., inj.

On the other hand, several diseases were reported to influence the pharmacokinetics of GCs. For example, dexamethasone clearance increased (165 %) and its half-life decreased (70 %) in renal failure (Kawai et al, 1985). This can be explained by decreased protein binding of dexamethasone to albumin in uremia (Rosman et al., 1984). In patients with chronic liver disease, dexamethasone clearance decreased (65 %) and the half-life increased (170 %), probably due to changes in albumin levels (Kawai et al, 1985).

As pharmacodynamic interactions, co-administration of GCs with methylxanthines (e.g. theophylline), β_2-agonists, or co-incidence with smoking should be considered. Theophylline acting as a non-selective phosphodiesterase inhibitor and adenosin receptor antagonist has glucocorticoid-sparing effect in patients with asthma and chronic obstructive pulmonary disease (COPD) (Markham and Faulds, 1998). This effect is probably caused by enhanced histone deacetylase (HDAC) activity in endothelial cells and macrophages (Ito et al., 2002). Contrary, smoking reduces HDAC activity, leading to overexpression of inflammatory mediators in smokers and need of higher doses of GCs (Ito et al., 2001). GCs and β_2-agonists have synergistic effect in reducing cell proliferation in bronchial smooth muscle (Roth et al., 2002, Czock et al., 2005)]; GCs increase expression of β_2-receptors and thus prevent the tolerance to β_2-agonists.

It might be presumed that the effect of synthetic steroids varies according to their susceptibility to metabolism by 11β-HSDs and binding affinity for GR and MR. For example, dexamethasone is relatively resistent to 11β-HSDs and acts as a potent selective GR agonist, but prednisolone is relatively selective for GR over MR and is susceptible to metabolism by 11β-HSDs (Diederich et al. 2004).

In immune cells, expression of 11β-HSD enzymes is not completely understood. In *in vitro* studies, 11β-HSD1 was expressed upon differentiation of human monocytes to macrophages, while 11β-HSD2 was not detectable in either monocytes or cultured macrophages. Several cytokines, such as IL-4 and IL-13, up-regulate expression of 11β-HSD1, what may result in increased level of active intracellular cortisol and suppressed production of inflammatory mediators by macrophages (Thieringer et al. 2001)]. On the other hand, TNFα, IL-1β, or IL-6 failed to increase 11β-HSD1 activity in the monocytes, but TNFα and IL-1β induced 11β-HSD1 activity in human aortic and bronchial smooth muscle cells (Cai et al. 2001).

Mechanisms of Action of GCs

Genomic mechanisms of action of GCs

GCs mediate most of their effects genomically. As lipophilic agents, glucocorticoid molecules easily diffuse across the cell membrane and bind to GR receptors in the cytoplasm (*Figure 1/⓪*). Upon ligand binding, GR is activated and dissociated from a heat shock protein (hsp)-90 containing chaperone complex (Pratt et al. 2004) (*Figure 1/①*). Then, the activated GR rapidly translocate to the nucleus, whereas the translocation is promoted by nuclear import proteins, such as importin α (karyopherin β) (Goldfarb et al. 2004) and importin 13 (Tao et al. 2005). Once in the nucleus, DNA binding domain of GR directs binding and receptor dimerization on near DNA sequences, called simple glucocorticoid response elements (GREs) (Newton et al. 2000, Rhen and Cidlowski 2005). This interaction results in the *transactivation* of genes controlled by GREs and induction (or „switching-on") of anti-inflammatory genes expression. This mechanism directly modulates expression of anti-inflammatory cytokines IL-10 and TGFβ, secretory leukocyte proteinase inhibitor (SLPI), IL-1 receptor antagonist or C1q, and annexin 1 (or lipocortin 1) mediating many of anti-inflammatory actions of GCs (Barnes 1998, Czock et al. 2005, McColl et al. 2007).

Nevertheless, most of genes are regulated indirectly by GR via suppression of gene expression (or *transrepression*). Ligand-activated GR can „switch-off" expression of the inflammatory genes through protein-protein interactions with activated nuclear factor (NF)-κB and activator of protein (AP)-1 transcription factors, finally leading to suppressed synthesis of pro-inflammatory substances, such as cytokines (IL-1, IL-2, IL-6, IL-12, TNFα, GM-CSF), chemokines (IL-8, eotaxin, MIP-1α), pro-inflammatory enzymes (COX-2, $cPLA_2$, iNOS), or adhesion molecules (ICAM-1, E-selectin) (Czock et al. 2005, McColl et al. 2007). As higher concentrations of GCs are required for induction of anti-inflammatory gene expression than for gene repression, repression of pro-inflammatory transcription factors appears to be a dominant mechanism of GC action (McColl et al. 2007).

Additionally, GCs have potent inhibitory effects on mitogen-activated protein kinase (MAPK) signalling pathways through induction of MAPK phosphatase (MKP)-1. MKP-1 dephosphorylates and inactivates MAPKs, such as p38 MAPK and c-Jun terminal kinase (JNK), which contribute to enhanced expresssion of pro-inflammatory mediators (Abraham et al. 2006). GCs may suppress the inflammation also through post-transitional effects, as they enhance expression of proteins destabilizing mRNA of certain pro-inflammatory proteins, such as TNFα (Bergmann et al. 2004, Barnes 2010). However, there is an additional DNA binding-independent mechanism of GCs action - reversible alterations in chromatin structure and histone acetylation. This proces may be important for „switching-off" genes once the stimulus is removed and inflammation is no longer required (McColl et al. 2007).

Nongenomic mechanisms of action of GCs

In the mentioned genomically-mediated processes (*Figure 1/⓪*), transcription and translation with subsequent proteosynthesis require at least 30 minutes up to several hours or days until some changes may be observed (Goulding 2004). However, GCs act also through nongenomically-mediated mechanisms (*Figure 1/①②③*). These are responsible for rapid GCs action occuring within seconds to minutes (Stellato 2004). Interactions between genomic and nongenomic mechanisms have been claimed, thereby controlling genomic mechanisms through nongenomic ones (Wehling 1997). Nongenomic effects occur faster and may be clinically relevant over a limited period, „bridging the gap" until the genomic effects take place (Buttgereit et al. 1999).

GCs exert rapid effects on various tissues and cells modulating hormone secretion, neuronal excitability, carbohydrate metabolism, cell morphology, cell behaviour, and other processes within seconds or minutes (Falkenstein et al. 2000, Stellato 2004). GCs could diminish or prevent the acute immune response by interfering with processes such as rise in intracellular Ca^{2+} concentration (Buttgereit 2000), effects on inflammatory signal transduction cascades including MAPK, neutrophil degranulation, phagocytosis by macrophages, cellular adhesion or actin cytoskeleton (Stellato 2004, Long et al. 2005, Liu et al. 2005). GCs may nongenomically affect also cellular energy metabolism (Buttgereit and Scheffold 2002), neuronal activity (Chen and Qiu 2001), or the second messenger systems (Buttgereit and Scheffold 2002).

Rapid effects of GCs were demonstrated in many tissues, for example, effect of dexamethasone in endometrial cells (Koukouritaki et al. 1996), or corticosterone in vascular smooth muscle cells (Muto et al. 2000). In the respiratory system, dexamethasone produced a rapid decrease in intracellular Ca^{2+} and inhibited Ca^{2+}-dependent Cl^- secretion (Urbach et al. 2002), and modulated Na^+/H^+ exchange activity in bronchial epithelial cells (Verriére et al. 2005). GCs inhibited also the airway smooth muscle contraction, as was observed within 10 min after budesonide inhalation (Zhou et al. 2003, Sun et al. 2006). Recently, low concentrations of corticosterone rapidly increased a production of superoxide anions by macrophages, as an immunopermissive effect (Shi et al. 2011).

In literature, several possible nongenomic mechanisms are discussed, such as specific interaction with the cytosolic GR receptor and successive release of hsp-90 and special proteins Src and MAPK (*Figure 1/①*), or specific interactions with membrane-bound glucocorticoid receptors (*Figure 1/③*) [Buttgereit and Scheffold 2002]. However, some immediate GCs effects may be GR independent (*Figure 1/②*), e.g. inhibition of superoxide production by macrophages (Long et al. 2005), or interactions with cell membranes (Buttgereit and Scheffold 2002).

Thus, GCs have three distinct therapeutically relevant effects (genomic, specific nongenomic, and unspecific nongenomic). Genomic effects are mediated by cytosolic receptors that alter expression of specific genes. Specific nongenomic effects occur within a few minutes and are mediated by steroid-selective membrane receptors. Unspecific nongenomic effects occur within seconds, but only at high GCs dosages, and seem to result from direct interactions with biological membranes (Buttgereit 2000). Thus, the hypothesis arised that the relative potencies of nongenomic and genomic effects of GCs may differ (Buttgereit et al. 1999). Buttgereit et al. (1999) measured the immediate unspecific nongenomic potencies of five clinically important GCs on respiration, on protein synthesis, and on Na^+-K^+-ATPase and Ca^{2+}-ATPase in concanavalin A-stimulated rat thymocytes and found a hierarchy (prednylidene 3.0 > dexamethasone 1.2 > methylprednisolone 1.0 > prednisolone 0.4 > betamethasone 0.2) completely different from that for the classical effects. Similar hierarchy was obtained also in evaluation of immediate effects of the mentioned GCs on cellular energy metabolism in quiescent peripheral blood mononuclear cells (Schmid et al. 2000).

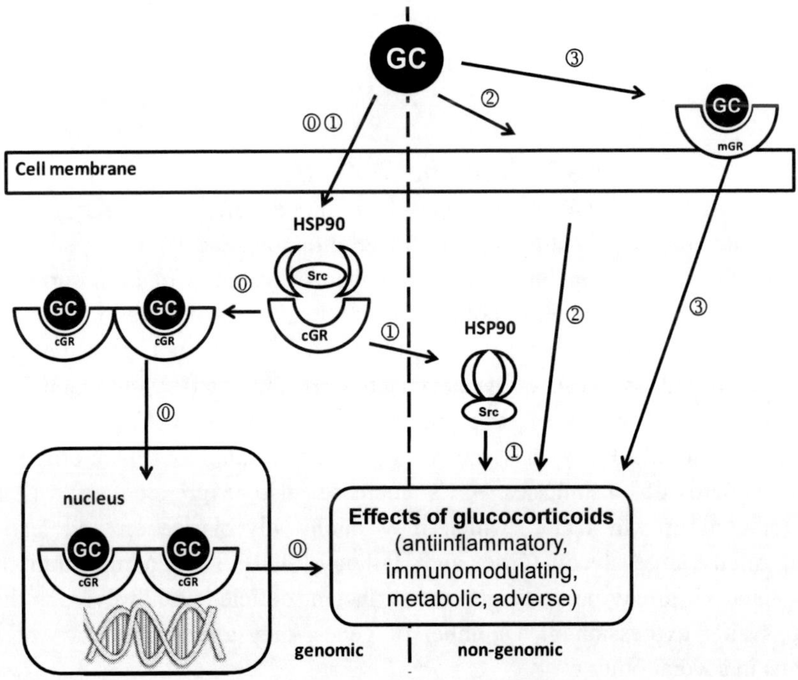

Figure 1. Mechanism of action of glucocorticoids. *GC*, glucocorticoid; *cGR*, cytoplasmic GC receptor; *mGR*, membrane-bound GC receptor; *HSP90*, heat shock protein 90; *Src*, protein. For explanations (⓪, ①, ②, and ③) see the text. (Adapted from Buttgereit et al., 2004; Stahn et al., 2007; Mokra and Mokry, 2011).

These data suggest why the clinical effect of, for instance, dexamethasone and betamethasone may differ despite their similar affinities for nuclear receptors. Furthermore, these findings show that a classical expression of clinical potency of individual GCs according to the ability to suppress cortisol production does not reflect sufficiently an ability, for instance, to suppress inflammation, which is significantly mediated also through the nongenomic mechanisms (Dubois 2005).

Irrespective of mechanisms of their action, GCs effectively suppress inflammation, lung edema formation, and pulmonary vasoconstriction. In addition, GCs act as important regulators of apoptosis and phagocytic removal of apoptotic cells, and thereby influence resolution of inflammation (McColl et al. 2007). GCs may have apoptotic or anti-apoptotic effects, depending on the cell type. For example, GCs increase the rate of apoptosis in eosinophils, what is important in attenuation of the inflammatory response, e.g. in asthma. On the other hand, GCs decrease the rate of apoptosis in neutrophils what might explain a limited efficacy of GCs in COPD, where the neutrophilic inflammation prevails (Czock et al. 2005).

Administration of GCs in the perinatal period

During the final prenatal period of fetal lung development in humans, GCs accelerate lung cell maturation and differentiation, and stimulate surfactant production in the fetal lungs, as they enhance synthesis of both surfactant-associated proteins and phospholipids, and increase rate of secretion (Creuwels et al. 1997, Isohama and Rooney 2001). GCs induce not only the genes associated with synthesis of surfactant proteins, fatty acid synthase, epithelial sodium channel and membrane protein sodium/potassium ATPase, but also several antioxidant enzymes including catalase, glutathione peroxidase and two superoxide dismutases. GCs increase also expression of vascular endothelial growth factor, which may inhibit alveolarization and lead to abnormally large alveoli (Grier and Halliday 2004). Thus, administration of antenatal GCs may partially prevent surfactant deficiency, however, as these drugs alter expression of a number of genes, they affect maturation of the lungs in several other ways.

The use of both antenatal and postnatal GCs has increased in the past decade. Antenatal GCs (particularly dexamethasone and betamethasone) have to accelerate lung maturation and stimulate synthesis and secretion of surfactant. In the studies by Beers et al. (1995) and Ramin et al. (2004), dexamethasone enhanced expression of pulmonary surfactant protein B (SP-B), which stimulates formation of phospholipid film *in vitro* and is essential for normal surfactant function *in vivo*. Similarly, maternal administration of betamethasone elevated SP-A protein and SP-A/SP-B mRNA levels in rabbit fetal lung tissue (Durham et al. 1993) and dose-dependently increased concentrations of saturated phosphatidylcholine (Ballard et al. 1997). Dexamethasone acts directly on type II cells to enhance the response to surfactant secretagogues and the effect is mediated by GR receptor (Isohama and Rooney 2001). Postnatally, GCs (particularly dexamethasone) are used in the treatment of consequences and complications in the premature newborns, such as bronchopulmonary dysplasia or chronic lung disease. Systemic GCs reduce activation of neutrophils and macrophages and decrease concentrations of inflammatory markers (Wang et al. 1997, Nupponen et al. 2002, Aghai et al. 2006). Moreover, GCs may enhance lung compliance and resistance and may finally improve the gas exchange in ventilator-dependent infants (Sanders et al. 1994, Bancalari 1998, Durand et al. 2002, Suchomski and Cummings 2002) and lower incidence of bronchopulmonary dysplasia (Rastogi et al. 1996, Yeh et al. 1997). However, in some studies use of GCs did not modify mortality or incidence of bronchopulmonary dysplasia (Tapia et al. 1998). Even, treatment of preterm infants with repeated and/or high doses of GCs may evoke long-term side effects on somatic, cerebral, and lung growth (Yeh et al. 1998, Shinwell et al. 2000, Bolt et al. 2001, Anttila et al. 2005). As shown in experimental studies on rats, antenatal and postnatal dexamethasone treatment may impair normal postnatal lung growth and increase the risk for pulmonary hypertension (Le Cras et al. 2000, Okajima et al. 2001). Thus, the balance between short-term gain and possible long-term side effects of glucocorticoids in preterms remains a difficult issue (Bolt et al. 2001).

Glucocorticoids in the treatment of MAS

Effect of the treatment depends on specific pharmacological properties, dose, and mode of delivery of the individual GCs, as well as on current status of the newborn or experimental animal with MAS, concomitant diseases etc. Different properties of individual GCs are related to different mineral-ocorticoid activity and potency to suppress cortisol production, and to potency of their nongenomic action. For example, potency of dexamethasone was superior to other tested GCs, probably thanks to the lowest lipophilicity, that enables direct interaction with the cell membrane (Buttgereit et al. 1999, Lösel and Wehling 2003).

In the animal models and in the newborns with MAS, several GC preparations have been used, e.g. hydrocortisone, prednisolone, methyl-prednisolone, and budesonide. For example, repeated administration of *hydrocortisone* had significant effect neither on the lung functions in newborn rabbits (Frantz et al. 1975), nor in neonates with MAS (Yeh et al. 1977). Instillation of high-dose *prednisolone* showed superior effect on lung histology and gas exchange to the standard dose, but potentiated oxidation stress in puppies with MAS (Kirimi et al. 2003). In a porcine model of MAS, pretreatment with *methylprednisolone* 30 minutes before instillation of meconium tended to prevent an early increase in pulmonary artery pressure and inhibited the second phase progressive rise in pulmonary artery pressure and pulmonary vascular resistance, decreased venous admixture and formation of lung edema and improved oxygenation (Soukka et al. 1997). In newborns with MAS, methylprednisolone administered for a period of 7 days shortened a period of oxygen delivery and duration of hospital stay, improved radiological clearance of the lungs and decreased levels of TNFα in the tracheal aspirate (Basu et al. 2007, Tripathi and Saili 2007, Tripathi et al. 2007). In meconium-instilled rabbits, *budesonide* administered intratracheally using an inpulsion effect of high-frequency jet ventilation effectively alleviated inflammation, diminished lung edema formation and meconium-induced tracheal and lung airway hyperreactivity to histamine, improved gas exchange and decreased oxidative injury of the lungs compared with non-treated controls (Mokra et al. 2007ab, Mokra et al. 2008b). In newborns with MAS, budesonide given for a period of 7 days shortened a period of oxygen delivery and duration of hospital stay and improved radiological clearance of the lungs, while no serious adverse effects were found (Basu et al. 2007, Tripathi and Saili 2007, Tripathi et al. 2007). Nevertheless, *dexamethasone* is the most often used GC preparation in the treatment of MAS at the moment.

Dexamethasone

Pharmacological properties of dexamethasone

Dexamethasone (9α-fluoro-16α-methylprednisolone, *Figure 2*) is a representative of long-term acting synthetic GCs. Due to lipophilic character similar to other GCs, dexamethasone is administered as a prodrug, when given intravenously.

Dexamethasone has potent anti-inflammatory and immunosuppressive effects. It is about 30-times stronger than hydrocortisone and about 5-times stronger than prednisone (Katzung et al. 2012). Generally, its pharmacological effects are based on mechanism of action of glucocorticosteroids and by comparing with other GCs, both pharmacokinetic and pharmacodynamic properties should be taken into consideration (*Table 2*).

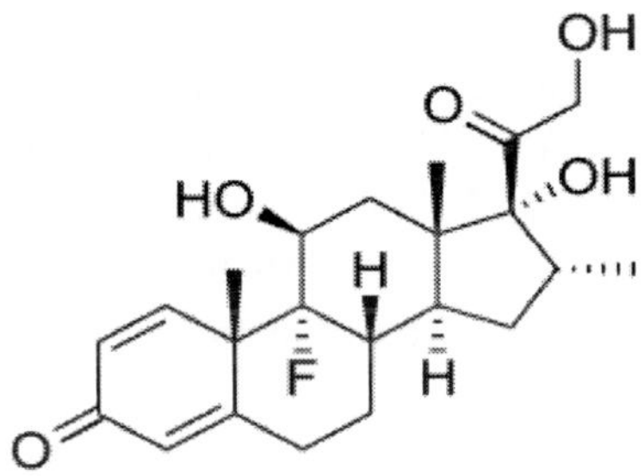

Figure 2. Molecular structure of dexamethasone (http://en.wiktionary.org/wiki/File: Dexamethasone_structure.svg).

Effects of Dexamethasone in MAS

In vitro studies

In *in vitro* studies, dexamethasone effectively inhibited a meconium-induced overproduction of NO (Li et al. 2001, Khan et al. 2002b)] and down-regulated expression of iNOS (Li et al. 2001, Kytola et al. 2003), COX-2 (Kytola et al. 2003), and thromboxane A_2 (Khan et al. 2002c).

Experimental studies

Several experimental and clinical studies evaluated efficacy and management of dexamethasone delivery in the conditions of MAS. Commonly, a dexamethasone dose of 0.5 mg/kg body weight of dexamethasone has been established. Nevertheless, timing of dexamethasone administration appeared to be critical for effectiveness of the treatment.

In 10-12 days-old piglets, pretreatment with dexamethasone (given 1 hour before meconium instillation) significantly prevented a meconium-induced rise in the pulmonary pressure and pulmonary vascular resistance and improved oxygenation expressed as PaO_2/FiO_2, but no significant effect on oxygenation and pulmonary hemodynamics was observed when dexamethasone was given 1 hour after meconium instillation (Holopainen et al. 2001). In a histological examination of the lung tissue, a prophylactic dexamethasone administration tended to decrease the severity of the pulmonary inflammatory changes, but there was no clear effect on the lung histology found in the group of animals treated 1 hour after meconium. On the other hand, both the prophylactic and "1-hour-after" dexamethasone administrations decreased the number of apoptotic cells, which were increased under the influence of meconium (Holopainen et al. 2001). Both treatments prevented a meconium-induced fall in the amount of blood leukocytes, and resulted in a marked increase in their number from 3 hours on, especially after prophylactic dexamethasone. However, neither the prophylactic administration nor administration of dexamethasone 1 hour after meconium instillation did reduce significantly the lung edema formation or lung tissue PLA_2 activity in piglets (Holopainen et al. 2001).

In a rabbit model of MAS, an early administration of dexamethasone (30 min after meconium instillation) tended to prevent a meconium-induced decrease in total blood leukocytes, increased a number of circulating neutrophils and showed the trend to decrease circulating eosinophils in the arterial blood at 5 hours of the treatment administration compared to non-treated meconium-instilled animals (Mokry et al. 2006). In the bronchoalveolar lavage fluid examined at the end of experiments, lower count of neutrophils and slightly lower count of eosinophils was observed after the treatment. In addition, dexamethasone suppressed a meconium-induced hyperreactivity of the tracheal smooth muscle and lung tissue to histamine, whereas no significant changes in the airway reactivity were observed in response to acetylcholine (Mokry et al. 2006).

Regarding these pilot results suggesting the benefit of dexamethasone treatment on inflammation in a rabbit model of MAS, our following study compared effects of one and two doses of dexamethasone, whereas the first one was given 30 min after meconium instillation and the second one was given two hours later. This approach was based on our observation that the lung function parameters are going to worsen from 2-3 hours of dexamethasone administration. It results from fast, but relatively short-term action of dexamethasone, with plasma half-time in adults about 190 min. Therefore, dexamethasone might be administered repetitively every 2-4 hours (data given by producer, Dexamed, Medochemie Cyprus). Both treatments, i.e. single-dose dexamethasone and two-dose dexamethasone reduced the lung edema formation expressed as a wet-dry weight ratio and decreased total number of cells and percentage of neutrophils in the bronchoalveolar lavage fluid (*Figure 4A and 4B*), which was associated with an increase in both circulating total leukocytes and neutrophils in the arterial blood (Mokra et al. 2007c) (*Figure 3A and 3B*). Dexamethasone decreased also the number of circulating eosinophils and reduced production of eosinophil cationic protein

(ECP) (Mokra et al. unpublished observation) (*Figure 5A and 5B*). Furthermore, both treatment regimen suppressed the meconium-induced tracheal hyperresponsiveness to histamine, and decreased concentrations of products of lipid peroxidation (thiobarbituric acid-reactive substances, TBARS) and protein oxidation (dityrosines, lysine-lipoperoxidation products) in the lung homogenate compared with non-treated controls (*Figure 6A, B, and 7A*), whereas all the mentioned changes were more obvious in two-dose dexamethasone treatment (Mokra et al. 2007c). Mitigation of oxidative stress in the lung tissue was detected also on the systemic level, where lower concentrations of TBARS and higher total antioxidant status (TAS) in the blood plasma were found (Mokra et al. unpublished observation) (*Figure 7B and 8A*). In the lung function parameters, dexamethasone treatment decreased central venous pressure and improved right-to-left pulmonary shunting, oxygenation index, $PaCO_2$, and pH in the arterial blood, what resulted into better ventilation efficiency index and reduced ventilatory pressures, with more pronounced effect observed in the two-dose dexamethasone (Mokra et al. 2008a).

In newborn piglets (5 days of age), dexamethasone at a dose of 0.5 mg/kg was delivered at 2 and 8 hours after meconium instillation, or animals received a normal saline at similar times (Khan et al. 1999). Within 4 hours, administration of the first dose of dexamethasone resulted in lower oxygen requirements, lower oxygenation index and $PaCO_2$, and significantly improved ventilatory efficiency index and lung compliance compared with non-treated controls. However, no additional improvement was observed after administration of the second dose of dexamethasone (Khan et al. 1999). Whereas no overt differences in the degree of inflammation or atelectasis were found in histological examination of the lungs (Khan et al. 1999), absence of clear effect on local inflammation, surfactant, and lung tissue injury in this study might be attributable to late administration of dexamethasone (2 hours after meconium instillation), when the meconium-induced inflammation has been already developed.

In newborn piglets (1-7 days old), dexamethasone sodium phosphate 0.5 mg/kg was given intravenously in two doses (with 12 hours time interval between the administrations). Piglets were further mechanically ventilated and tracheal aspirate samples were obtained, and several respiratory and cardiovascular parameters were daily monitored for 4 days. Dexamethasone treatment decreased concentrations of leukotrienes LTC4 and LTD4 and 6-keto$PGF_1\alpha$ in the tracheal aspirate when compared to the non-treated MAS group (Wu et al. 1999).

These results have clearly shown a superior effect of early administration of dexamethasone before generation of extensive inflammatory response to the meconium instillation. Nevertheless, limitations of the treatment efficacy in the late administration of GCs may be partially reduced by a repetitive administration.

Clinical studies

Paralel to experimental studies, effects of dexamethasone were studied also in the patients with MAS. In 27 newborns with severe MAS, dexamethasone was given every 12 hours in gradually decreasing doses for total 7 days (initial dose immediately after the diagnosis of MAS 1.0 mg/kg/dose, day 1-3: 0.5 mg/kg/dose, day 4-7: 0.25 mg/kg/dose). Such therapy lowered values of $PaCO_2$ and pH and facilitated weaning from the ventilator in the comparable ventilator settings and FiO_2/PaO_2.

On the other hand, there were no differences in mortality, chronic lung disease morbidity, duration of oxygen therapy, or duration of hospitalization (Wu et al. 1999). In a pilot clinical study, dexamethasone divided into two doses was given up to a maximum of 9 days in gradually decreasing doses (at a total dose of 0.5, 0.25, and 0.125 mg/kg/day, each dosing given for 3 days) in newborns with severe MAS (with oxygenation index >25) (da Costa et al. 2001). Despite the mean age of commencing dexamethasone was relatively high (79.9 hours), a significant improvement in oxygenation index was observed already at 8 hours, and then at following intervals at 16, 24, 32 and 40 hours compared with an initial time point.

Improvement in the respiratory status was observed in 13 of total 14 neonates with MAS, allowing weaning from the ventilator and eventual extubation at a mean age of 8.7 days. Unfortunately, the study by da Costa et al. (2001) was not carried out as a randomised controlled study and there was no control group.

There is a lack of information on administration of dexamethasone later then one week after the meconium aspiration. Nevertheless, even "late" dexamethasone may show some benefit. Dexamethasone delivered on the 10th day of age improved the lung functions in the newborn with severe MAS, who was previously not improving on the conventional therapy. Follow-up at 1 year of age showed normal psychomotor development and complete normalization of the chest X-ray (van den Anker and van Loenen 1994). Thus, dexamethasone may effectively modify also the late processes and complications associated with MAS, such as artificial ventilation-induced injury etc.

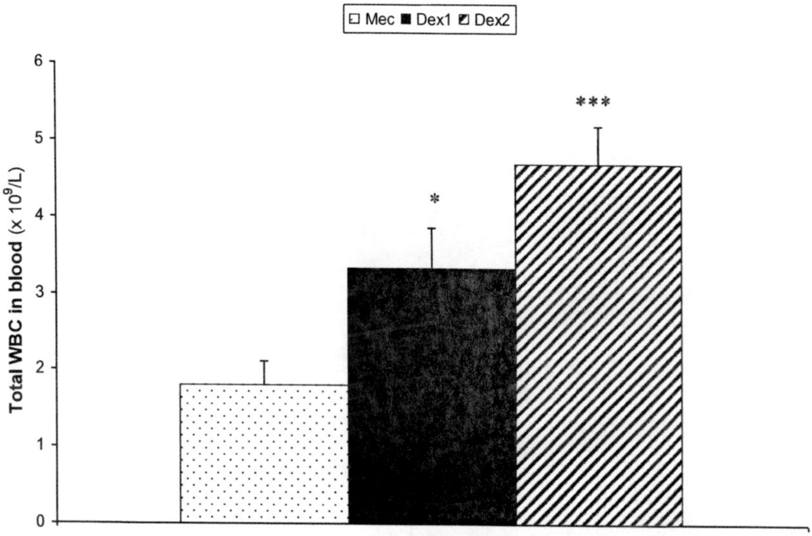

A

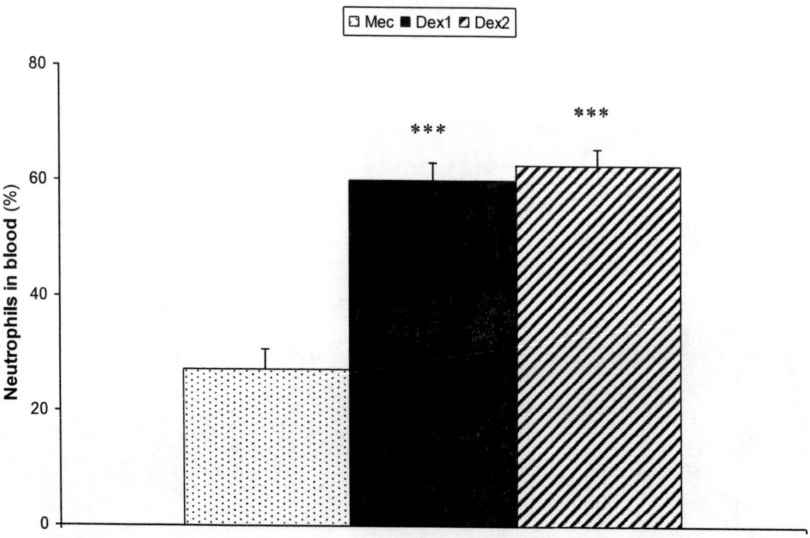

B

Figure 3. A. Total white blood cells (WBC) count in the blood (x 10^9/L). (Mokra et al. unpublished observation). B. Percentage of neutrophils in the blood (in %). (Adapted from Mokra et al. 2007c). For statistical differences between meconium-instilled non-treated animals (Mec) vs. meconium-instilled and single-dose dexamethasone-treated animals (Dex1) and vs. meconium-instilled and two-dose dexamethasone-treated animals (Dex2): $^{*}P$<0.05, $^{***}P$<0.001.

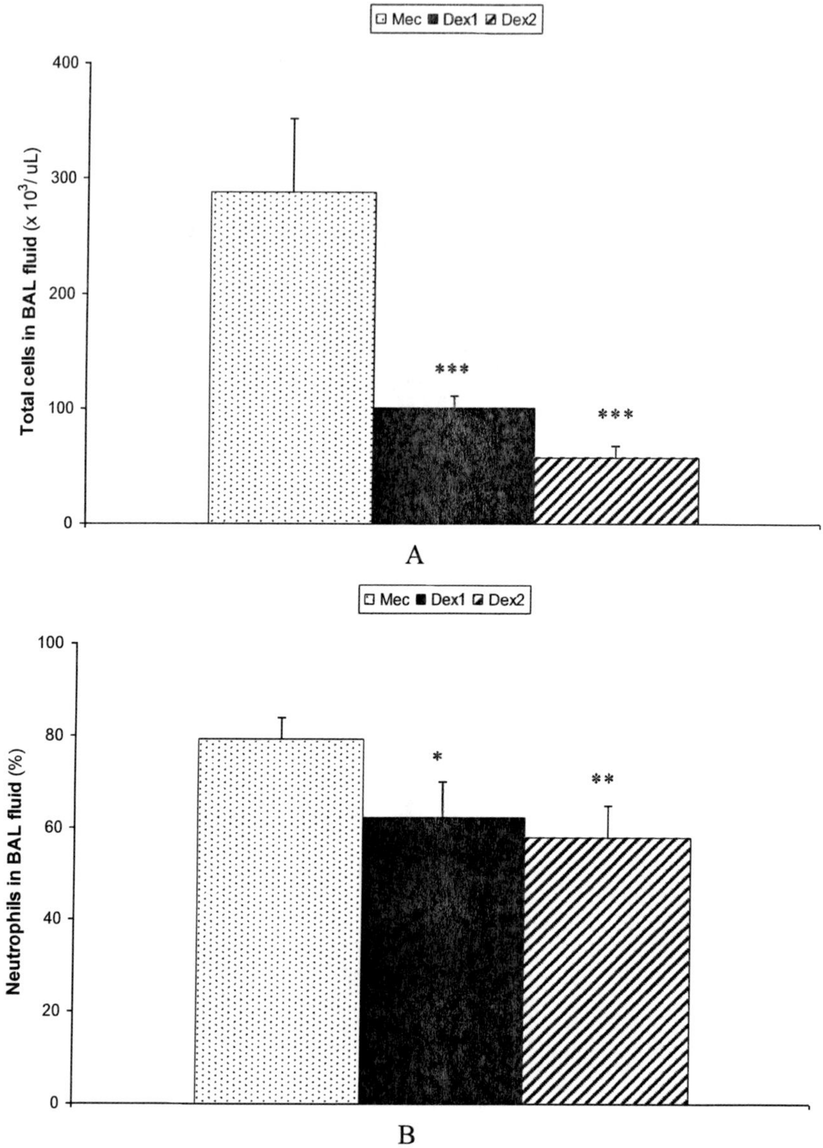

Figure 4. A. Total number of cells in the bronchoalveolar lavage (BAL) fluid (x 10^3/μL). B. Percentage of neutrophils in the BAL fluid (in %). For statistical differences between meconium-instilled non-treated animals (Mec) vs. meconium-instilled and single-dose dexamethasone-treated animals (Dex1) and vs. meconium-instilled and two-dose dexamethasone-treated animals (Dex2): $^{*}P<0.05$, $^{**}P<0.01$, $^{***}P<0.001$. (Adapted from Mokra et al. 2007c).

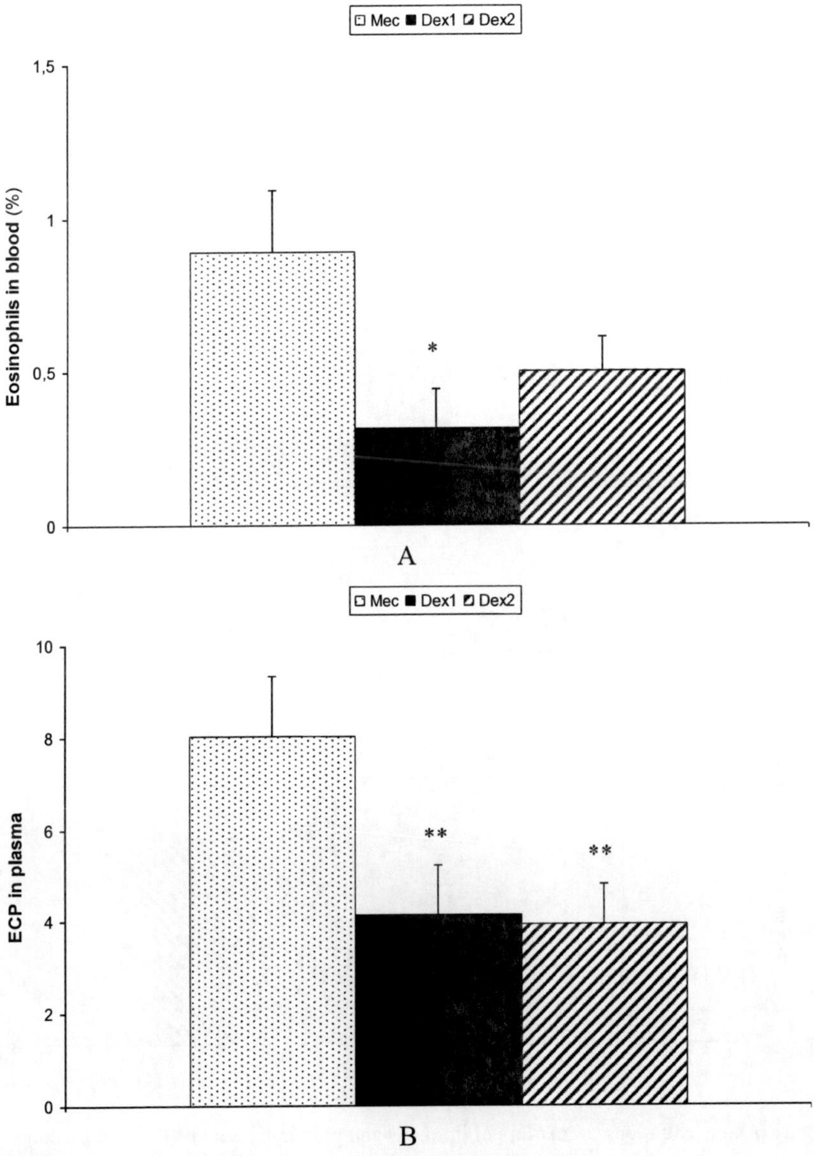

Figure 5. A. Percentage of eosinophils in the blood (in %). B. Concentration of eosinophil cationic protein (ECP) in the blood plasma (in μg/L). For statistical differences between meconium-instilled non-treated animals (Mec) vs. meconium-instilled and single-dose dexamethasone-treated animals (Dex1) and vs. meconium-instilled and two-dose dexamethasone-treated animals (Dex2): $^{*}P<0.05$, $^{**}P<0.01$. (Mokra et al. unpublished observation).

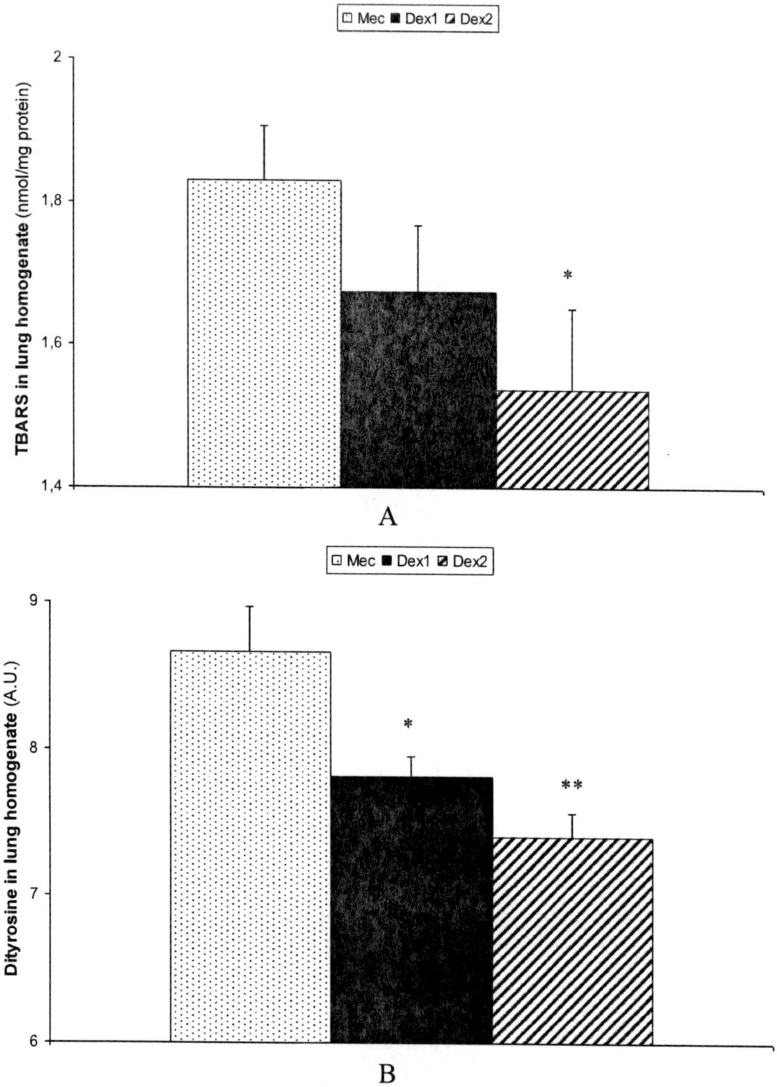

Figure 6. Concentrations of markers of lipid (A) and protein oxidation (B, C) in the lung homogenate. A. Thiobarbituric acid-reactive substances (TBARS, in nmol/mg protein). B. Dityrosines (in arbitrary units, A.U.). For statistical differences between meconium-instilled non-treated animals (Mec) vs. meconium-instilled and single-dose dexamethasone-treated animals (Dex1) and vs. meconium-instilled and two-dose dexamethasone-treated animals (Dex2): $^{*}P<0.05$, $^{**}P<0.01$. (Adapted from Mokra et al. 2007c).

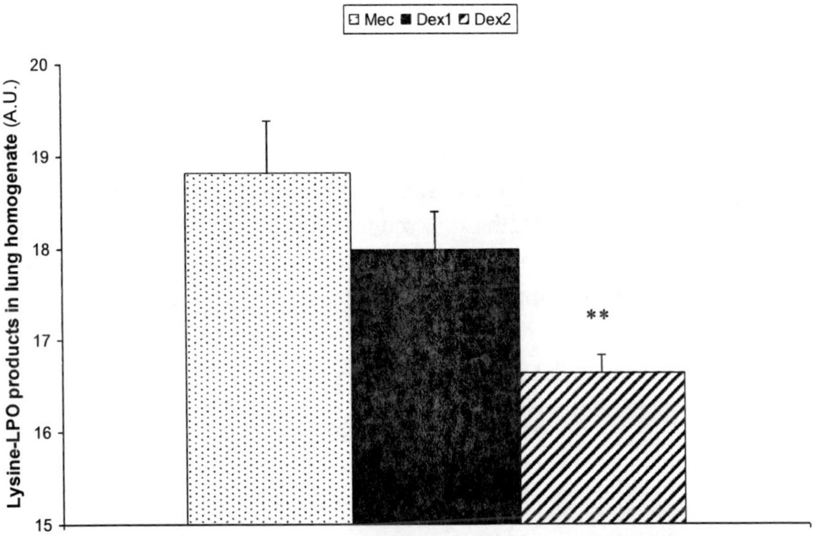

A

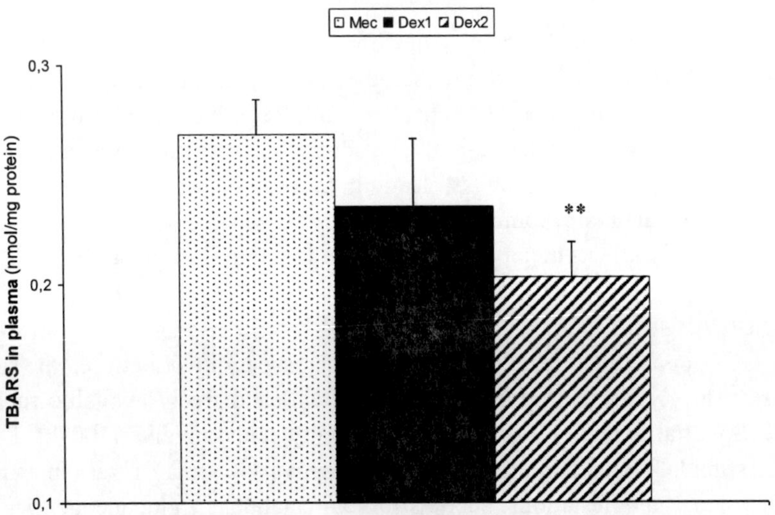

B

Figure 7. A. Lysine-lipoperoxidation (LPO) products (in arbitrary units, A.U.). B. Concentration of a marker of lipid oxidation – thiobarbituric acid-reactive substances (TBARS, in nmol/mg protein) in the blood plasma. For statistical differences between meconium-instilled non-treated animals (Mec) vs. meconium-instilled and single-dose dexamethasone-treated animals (Dex1) and vs. meconium-instilled and two-dose dexamethasone-treated animals (Dex2): $^{*}P<0.05$, $^{**}P<0.01$. (Mokra et al. unpublished observation).

Dexamethasone in animal models of the acute lung injury similar to MAS

Favourable results of dexamethasone administration were obtained also in the models of acute lung injury with features similar to MAS. Dexamethasone improved hemodynamics and pulmonary vascular remodelling in a monocrotaline-induced pulmonary arterial hypertension and improved survival in rats. Furthermore, dexamethasone reduced pulmonary IL-6 overexpression and IL-6-expressing inflammatory cell infiltration, and proliferation of rat pulmonary artery smooth muscle cells *in vitro* (Price et al. 2011). In rats with lung contusion, dexamethasone decreased a number of neutrophils in the BAL fluid, and reduced concentrations of oxidative stress markers, such as malonyldialdehyde and products of NO (nitrite/nitrate), and improved gas exchange (Türüt et al. 2009).

Side Effects of GCs in MAS

Side effects of GCs occur with different prevalence, in different organs, and after different duration of the therapy, and may occur as single or multiple adverse effects of the therapy (Schäcke et al. 2002). As stress hormones, GCs released via the hypothalamic-pituitary-adrenal axis recruit glucose to supply energy to organs facing stress, leading to arousal reactions and immune responses to maintain homeostasis. Failure to keep ample concentrations of GCs adversely affects metabolism and organ function (Lee et al. 2012).

Hyperglycemia

GCs oppose the effects of insulin and increase turnover between the stored energy (in glycogen, triglycerides and protein) and freely available fuel for mitochondrial oxidation (glucose and free fatty acids) (Walker 2007b). Long-term stimulation or administration of excessive GCs may result in various pathological manifestations, such as protein catabolism, gluconeogenesis and glycogenolyis, resulting in hyperglycemia in patients without known diabetes (induction of diabetes) and worsened glycemic control in diabetic patients (aggravation of diabetes). Excess of GCs causes both decreased β-cell insulin production and insulin resistance (Andrews and Walker 1999, Schäcke et al. 2002).

As in MAS studies GCs are used in a single dose or their administration lasts maximally several days, only transient hyperglycemia (not requiring therapy) was observed in several neonatal patients, and glycemia was normalized after reducing the dose of dexamethasone (Wu et al. 1999, da Costa et al. 2001). In a rabbit model of MAS, no significant changes in the blood glucose between the dexamethasone-treated and non-treated groups were observed, as well (Mokra et al. unpublished observation). These findings are in accordance with a previously published information, that the effects of GCs on hyperglycemia usually remit within 48 hours of discontinuation of GCs therapy (Schäcke et al. 2002).

Cardiovascular changes

GCs affect also the cardiovascular system: cause hypertension and dyslipidemia, and reduce the fibrinolytic potential. The mechanisms of GCs-induced hypertension are complex and include increase in systemic vascular resistence, extracellular volume, and cardiac contractility (Schäcke et al. 2002). Blood pressure in humans is subjected to a strict control by several systems, such as baroreceptors, natriuretic peptides, renin-angiotensin-aldosterone system, kinin-kallikrein system, adrenergic receptor system, nitric oxide, endothelin etc., which interact together in a complex fashion (Lifton et al. 2001).

Most of the cardiovascular side effects are mediated via GR or MR receptors, as both types of receptors are expressed in cardiovascular tissues including the heart and arterial walls. GCs act directly to maintain vascular tone and modify vascular inflammatory, proliferative, and remodelling responses to injury (Ullian 1999, Walker 2007b). Synthetic GCs, which bind to both GR and MR receptors and are not metabolized by 11β-HSDs, can cause hypertension by regulating epithelial Na^+ channels (ENaC) via MR. However, dexamethasone has no or little MR activity, so this mechanism of inducing hypertension seems to be of low importance.

On the other hand, attenuation of sympathetic nerve activity responses by GCs is thought to eliminate a positive feed-back effect of stress on sympathetic outflow. However, with a baroreceptor reflex, attenuation of reflex control of sympathetic nerve activity by GCs could be detrimental by contributing to the maintenance of hypertension produced by GCs or by other mechanisms (Scheuer and Mifflin 2001). In addition, GCs potentiate the central actions of angiotensin to increase arterial pressure (Scheuer and Bechtold 2001). However, adverse effects of GCs appear more likely after the long-term treatment, but less-frequently after the short-term treatment, even with high GCs doses. It might be explained by time-dependent genomic effects of GCs, which do not elevate further after high doses, when GR saturation is already achieved (Frauman 1996, Czock et al. 2005).

In addition to genomically-mediated effects, dexamethasone exerts potent nongenomic action, as mentioned in the previous subsection. Thus, some cardiovascular effects, particularly those occuring within several minutes, seem to be attributable to the nongenomic action of dexamethasone. Despite the acute cardiovascular changes may be critical for neonates with the meconium-induced lung injury, there is a lack of information on evaluation of adverse effects of GCs administration in neonatal MAS. This fact has inspired us to measure some cardiovascular parameters to validate objectively how serious might be the changes of cardiovascular parameters related to systemic GCs administration.

In our pilot study, slight changes in the blood pressure and heart rate in dexamethasone-treated vs. non-treated meconium-instilled animals were observed, but due to a small number of animals included in the groups the changes were not significant (Mokra et al. 2009). In continuation of these experiments, blood pressure tended to increase, heart rate decreased and some parameters of heart rate variability (expressing the activity of parasympathetic cardiac control) increased, whereas more obvious cardiovascular changes were observed in administration of two doses of dexamethasone than in a single-dose administration (Mokra et al. 2008a).

To evaluate these changes more in detail, a following study analyzed the changes in blood pressure, heart rate, and heart rate variability in dexamethasone-treated vs. non-treated meconium-instilled rabbits as well as in dexamethasone-treated or non-treated saline-instilled rabbits, which served as sham controls. Particular attention was paid to the changes in parameters of heart rate variability, which are sensitive markers of cardiovascular reactivity and parasympathetic autonomic control of the cardiac activity (Moguilevski et al. 1996, Task Force of the European Society of Cardiology and the North American Society of Pacing and Electrophysiology 1996). The cardiovascular changes were observed during 5 min of slow intravenous dexamethasone administration (or saline instillation in sham-controls) and during 5 min immediately after the period of treatment administration, as well as during 5 hours of the treatment administration in all groups of animals. The results showed increased blood pressure, decreased heart rate, increased heart rate variability and higher occurence of cardiac arrhythmias during and immediately after dexamethasone administration, while decreased heart rate and increased parameters of heart rate variability were observed till the end of the observation period (i.e. 5 hours after the first dose of dexamethasone) (Mokra et al. 2008c) (*Figure 8B*). Increased mean arterial blood pressure after intravenous dexamethasone administration was demonstrated also in the meconium-instilled piglets, where the difference to the non-treated group was significant at 2, 4 and 5 hours after dexamethasone administration. In the corresponding time intervals, systemic vascular resistence also slightly increased, however, differences to the non-treated group were not significant (Holopainen et al. 2001). In the newborns, administration of dexamethasone stabilized cardiovascular parameters, when transient elevation in blood pressure was noted on days 3-7 compared to dexamethasone non-treated newborns, whereas no differences between the groups were found in parameters measured by color Doppler echocardiography, such as pulmonary arterial pressure, pulmonary acceleration time (PAT)/ejection time (ET) ratio, or pre-ejection time (PET)/ET ratio (Wu et al. 1999). In the study by da Costa et al. (2001), no meconium-aspirated infants required treatment for hypertension; however, decelerating of the heart rate was seen in several infants after commencing dexamethasone.

On the other hand, no significant differences in the blood pressure and heart rate were observed between the dexamethasone-treated and non-treated control groups of meconium-instilled animals (Khan et al. 1999, Wu et al. 1999). Similarly, no changes in the blood pressure were found between the groups of newborns with severe MAS treated with standard therapy, BAL with exogenous surfactant and surfactant BAL combined with previous single-dose dexamethasone (Salvia-Roiges et al. 2004).

Some cardiovascular changes were observed after intravenous dexamethasone also in the saline-instilled controls, however, they were less obvious than those in the meconium-instilled animals (Mokra et al. 2008c). Similar acute cardiovascular effects of dexamethasone, i.e. increased systolic blood pressure and decreased heart rate as well as other changes, such as increased natriuretic peptide, decreased C-reactive protein, decreased aldosterone and tendency to attenuate NO-mediated vasodilation were previosly observed also in healthy volunteers (Brotman et al. 2005). We may presume a relationship between the cardiac autonomic regulation and inflammation or immune dysfunction (Gumprecht et al. 2002, Murray et al. 2003, Marsland et al. 2007). Contrary, in the study by Holopainen et al. (2001), dexamethasone had no effect on pulmonary or systemic hemodynamics in the ventilated piglets without meconium insult. However, cardiovascular parameters were firstly measured 15 min after administration of dexamethasone (Holopainen et al. 2001), when, as we can presume according to our findings, the most obvious changes in the blood pressure and heart rate have already disappeared.

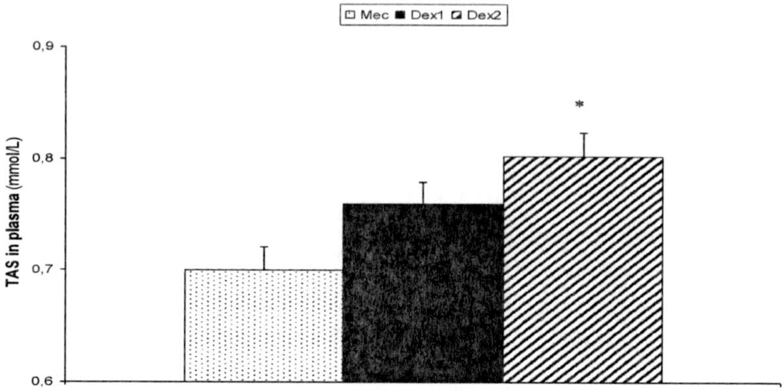

A

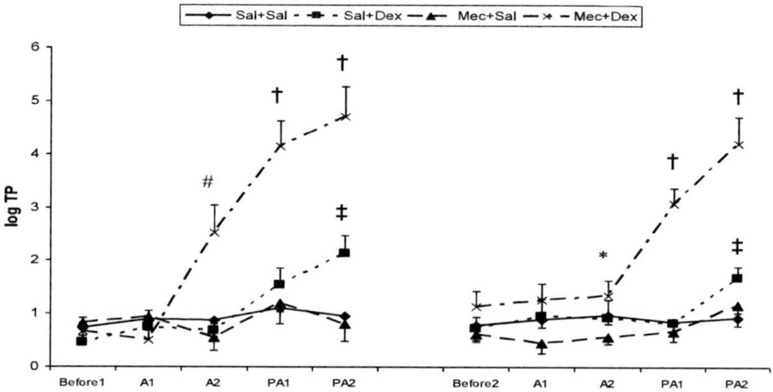

B

Figure 8. A. Total antioxidant status (TAS, in mmol/L) in the blood plasma. For statistical differences between meconium-instilled non-treated animals (Mec) vs. meconium-instilled and single-dose dexamethasone-treated animals (Dex1) and vs. meconium-instilled and two-dose dexamethasone-treated animals (Dex2): $^{*}P<0.05$, $^{**}P<0.01$. (Mokra et al. unpublished observation). B. Logarithm of total spectral power (log TP) during 5 min of intravenous administration of dexamethasone (or saline in sham-treated groups) (expressed in two intervals of 2.5 min, A1 and A2) and during 5 min immediately after the finishing the treatment administration (expressed in two intervals of 2.5 min, PA1 and PA2) in animals with intratracheal meconium instillation (Mec) treated by two doses of dexamethasone (Mec+Dex) or given saline instead of dexamethasone (sham-treated animals, Mec+Sal), and in animals with intratracheal saline instead of meconium (Sal, served as controls) treated by two doses of dexamethasone (Sal+Dex) or given saline instead of dexamethasone (sham-treated controls, Sal+Sal). Before 1, Before 2: before administration of the first dose (30 min after intratracheal meconium/saline) or the second dose (2 hours after the first dose) of the treatment, respectively. For statistical differences between: Mec+Dex vs. all other groups: $^{*}P<0.05$, $^{\#}P<0.01$, $^{\dagger}P<0.001$; Sal+Dex vs. Mec+Sal and Sal+Sal: $^{\ddagger}P<0.01$. (Adapted from Mokra et al. 2008c).

Other Side Effects

Systemic GCs (*Table 3*) may cause also hypokalemia, skin atrophy, dyslipidemia, reduced fibrinolysis, posterior subcapsular cataract, exacerbation of glaucoma, increased intracranial pressure, peptic ulcers, upper gastrointestinal bleeding, immunosuppression, neuropsychiatric disturbances, osteoporosis, myopathy, or irregularities of the menstruation cycle (Jantz and Sahn, 1999, Schäcke et al. 2002, Fernandes et al. 2005). However, these changes are more frequently observed after repetitive or long-term GCs administration. Because in MAS high-dose GCs are administered in a single or only in several doses, some acute adverse effects (e.g. cardiovascular), might be expected, but other effects e.g. on the metabolism are negligible.

Table 3. Side effects of GCs after systemic administration

System/organ	Side effects
Blood	Impaired fibrinolysis Thrombosis
Bone, muscles, fat tissue	Osteoporosis with increased risk of fractures Avascular necrosis of femoral head Fat redistribution (buffalo hump, increased abdominal fat) Thin arms and legs – muscle wasting myopathy Moon face with red plethoric cheeks Inhibition of growth
Cardiovascular system	Hypertension Cardiac hypertrophy Cardiac arrhythmias Increased vascular fragility
Central nervous system	Increased intracranial pressure (benign intracranial hypertension) Neuropsychiatric disturbances (euphoria, depression, psychotic symptoms, emotional lability) Abnormal neurological development
Eye	Posterior subcapsular cataract Exacerbation of glaucoma
Gastrointestinal system	Peptic ulcers Upper gastrointestinal bleeding
Immune system	Immunosuppression Increased susceptibility to infections (opportunistic infections)
Metabolism	Hyperglycemia Dyslipidemia Hypokalemia Negative nitrogen balance Increased appetite
Reproductive system	Irregularities of menstruation cycle
Skin	Thinning skin (skin atrophy) Poor wound healing Easy bruising

Nevertheless, in the newborns GCs should be used with a caution. In the term newborns with MAS, drop in weight was found several days after dexamethasone (Wu et al. 1999, da Costa et al. 2001), possibly attributed to loss of edema fluid or a true weight loss. Septicemia and infective pneumonia appeared sporadically (da Costa et al. 2001)]. In the preterm GCs-treated infants, short-term cardiovascular effects, such as hypertension and hypertrophic cardiomyopathy were described (Brand et al. 1993, Bensky et al. 1996, Skelton et al. 1998), and possible long-term neurological development alterations, such as cerebral palsy and/or delayed and abnormal neurological development (Yeh et al. 1998, Shinwell et al. 2000, Stark et al. 2001, Barrington 2001, Halliday 2001, Jones et al. 2005). Thus, despite no iatrogenic complications have been reported after treating full-term neonates or after a single dose of GCs, follow-up of the patients with MAS treated with GCs should include neurological and cardiovascular monitoring.

Dexamethasone in a Combination with Exogenous Surfactant

As mentioned above, surfactant dysfunction and inflammation are the principal pathomechanisms of MAS. Considering this, delivery of exogenous surfactant has become a major pharmacological approach in severe MAS. However, this treatment has little effect on meconium-induced inflammation.

Thus, it is reasonable to combine surfactant therapy with administration of anti-inflammatory agents, for instance, dexamethasone. Intravenous dexamethasone at a single dose of 0.5 mg/kg administered within the first 5 hours of life prior a bronchoalveolar lavage with diluted surfactant preparation beractant improved the status of eleven newborns with MAS more effectively than surfactant lavage alone (Salvia-Roiges et al. 2004). This combination led to a greater and more sustained improvement in oxygenation index at 24 and 48 hours of the treatment and reduced requirements for inhaled NO, oxygen therapy, mechanical ventilation, and hospitalization (Salvia-Roiges et al. 2004).

Other possibility is to add dexamethasone directly into a bolus of exogenous surfactant. Using surfactant as a vehicle, dexamethasone may suppress inflammation directly in the lungs, with less side effects. In a model of acute lung injury, intratracheal instillation of radiolabelled dexamethasone mixed with exogenous surfactant led to 10-fold higher concentrations of dexamethasone in the lung tissue than the intravenous administration. The intratracheal dexamethasone was well distributed throughout all four lobes of the lungs including the periphery (Nimmo et al. 2002). Similar distribution was observed when saline was used as a vehicle, however, delivery was more effective and consistent using the exogenous surfactant, without risk of abundant accumulation of water in the lungs or dilution of endogenous surfactant as it is in saline. In addition, systemic penetration of dexamethasone from the lungs to the circulation appeared to be slower when the drug was delivered in surfactant as opposed in saline (Nimmo et al. 2002), possibly due to enhanced solubilization of dexamethasone by the surfactant (Wiedmann et al. 2000). In the other model of acute lung injury, dexamethasone added to exogenous surfactant showed an additional improvement in gas exchange, ameliorating inflammation, and alleviating the lung tissue damage to surfactant-only treatment in rats (Chen et al. 2001).

Furthermore, dexamethasone could be administered topically in the form of aerosol. However, in such administration only a relatively small proportion of the drug reaches the lungs, and thereby has a limited success, particularly in the newborns (Merz et al. 1999, Nimmo et al. 2002).

Excessively high concentrations of GCs could impair the surfactant function, similarly to cholesterol. Nevertheless, no changes in the surface tension of undiluted artificial surfactant (Survanta) or in diluted Survanta in any of the used concentrations were observed after mixing with dexamethasone (Nimmo et al. 2002).

Perspectives of Optimized GCs and Selective Glucocorticoid Receptor Agonists in MAS

Administration of dexamethasone in MAS is usually short-term, ranging from a single-dose instillation to a dose-reducing protocol lasting several days. Despite this, several adverse effects of intravenous dexamethasone administration, particularly on cardiovascular parameters, may limit the usefulness of this treatment. Nevertheless, new variations of the conventional GCs have been recently introduced, such as nitro-steroids (Perretti et al. 2003, Paul-Clark et al. 2003), long circulating liposomal glucocorticoids (Schweingruber et al. 2011, Crielaard et al. 2011), and qualitatively new drugs called selective glucocorticoid receptor agonists (SEGRAs) (Stahn et al. 2007, Löwenberg et al. 2007, De Bosscher et al. 2010, De Bosscher 2010). These innovative steroidal or non-steroidal molecules induce transrepression, while transactivation is less affected (Stahn et al. 2007, Löwenberg et al. 2008, De Bosscher et al. 2010). Thanks to this, the mentioned drugs may have comparable or even superior anti-inflammatory effects to GCs, but with proposed less side effects. Optimized GCs and SEGRAs were successfully used in various diseases with inflammation feature (Paul-Clark et al. 2003, De Bosscher et al. 2008, Schweingruber et al. 2011). Thus, it is well appreciated that in the future optimized GCs and SEGRAs may be included also into the treatment protocol of the respiratory inflammatory diseases, such as MAS.

Conclusion

GCs are potent drugs with pleiotropic effects that are mediated by both genomic and nongenomic mechanisms. Regarding the complex pathophysiology of MAS with massive inflammation, lung edema and pulmonary vasoconstriction, administration of GCs may be beneficial also in the treatment of this serious neonatal disease. Within the last decades, several GCs preparations have been used in various experimental models and in the newborns with MAS. However, dexamethasone with its rapid action has become the most suitable choice in this indication. If given early, dexamethasone effectively suppresses meconium-induced inflammation, reduces accumulation of liquid in the lungs, and alleviates pulmonary hypertension, what finally results in an improvement in the lung functions. Therapeutic effect appears already after a single dose of dexamethasone, however, efficacy of the treatment potentiates in a repetitive administration. On the other hand, repetitive dexamethasone administration may be associated with higher occurance of side effects. Thus, possible benefits and risks of the treatment should be carefully considered with a particular respect to a general status of the newborn suffering from MAS.

Acknowledgments

This work was supported by the Project "Center of Excellence for Perinatology Research CEPV1 and CEPV2", co-financed from EU sources; by the Project of Slovak Research and Development Agency APVV-435-11; and by the Projects of Ministry of Education of Slovak Republic VEGA No. 1/0057/11 and No. 1/0030/11.

References

[No authors listed]. Heart rate variability: standards of measurement, physiological interpretation and clinical use. Task Force of the European Society of Cardiology and the North American Society of Pacing and Electrophysiology. *Circulation,* 1996, 93, 1043-1065.

Abraham, SM; Lawrence, T; Kleiman, A; Warden, P; Medghalchi, M; Tuckermann, J; Saklatvala, J; Clark, AR. Antiinflammatory effects of dexamethasone are partly dependent on induction of dual specificity phosphatase 1. *J Exp Med,* 2006, 203, 1883-1889.

Aghai, ZH; Kumar, S; Farhath, S; Kumar, MA; Saslow, J; Nakhla, T; Eydelman, R; Strande, L; Stahl, G; Hewitt, C; Nesin, M; Rahman, I. Dexamethasone suppresses expression of Nuclear Factor-kappaB in the cells of tracheobronchial lavage fluid in premature neonates with respiratory distress. *Pediatr Res,* 2006, 59, 811-815.

Andrews, RC; Walker, BR. Glucocorticoids and insulin resistence: old hormones, new targets. *Clin Sci,* 1999, 96, 513-523.

Anttila, E; Peltoniemi, O; Haumont, D; Herting, E; ter Horst, H; Heinonen, K; Kero, P; Nykänen, P; Oetomo, SB; Hallman, M. Early neonatal dexamethasone treatment for prevention of bronchopulmonary dysplasia. Randomised trial and meta-analysis evaluating the duration of dexamethasone therapy. *Eur J Pediatr,* 2005, 164, 472-481.

Asad, A; Bhat, R. Pharmacotherapy for meconium aspiration. *J Perinatol,* 2008, 28 Suppl 3, 72-78.

Avoine, O; Bossé, D; Beaudry, B; Beaulieu, A; Albadine, R; Praud, JP; Robert, R; Micheau, P; Walti, H. Total liquid ventilation efficacy in an ovine model of severe meconium aspiration syndrome. *Crit Care Med,* 2011, 39, 1097-1103.

Bacsik, RD. Meconium aspiration syndrome. *Pediatr Clin North Am,* 1977, 24, 463-479.

Ballard, PL; Ning, Y; Polk, D; Ikegami, M; Jobe, AH. Glucocorticoid regulation of surfactant components in premature lambs. *Am J Physiol,* 1997, 273, L1048-L1057.

Bancalari, E. Corticosteroids and neonatal chronic lung disease. *Eur J Pediatr,* 1998, 157, S31-S37.

Barnes, PJ. Anti-inflammatory actions of glucocorticoids: molecular mechanisms. *Clin Sci (Lond),* 1998, 94, 557-572.

Barnes, PJ. Mechanisms and resistance in glucocorticoid control of inflammation. *J Steroid Biochem Mol Biol,* 2010, 120, 76-85.

Barrington, KJ. The adverse neuro-developmental effects of postnatal steroids in the preterm infant: a systematic review of RCTs. *BMC Pediatr,* 2001, 1, 1.

Basu, S; Kumar, A; Bhatia, BD; Satya, K; Singh, TB. Role of steroids on the clinical course and outcome of meconium aspiration syndrome-a randomized controlled trial. *J Trop Pediatr,* 2007, 53, 331-337.

Beers, MF; Shuman, H; Liley, HG; Floros, J; Gonzales, LW; Yue, N; Ballard, PL. Surfactant protein B in human fetal lung: developmental and glucocorticoid regulation. *Pediatr Res,* 1995, 38, 668-675.

Bensky, AS; Kothadia, JM; Covitz, W. Cardiac effects of dexamethasone in very low birth weight infants. *Pediatrics,* 1996, 97, 818-821.

Bergmann, MW; Staples, KJ; Barnes, PJ; Newton, R. Nuclear factor-kappaB does not mediate the inhibitory effects of dexamethasone on granulocyte-macrophage colony-stimulating factor expression. *Immunology,* 2004, 111, 430-434.

Blackburn, ST; Loper, DL. *Maternal, fetal and neonatal physiology.* Philadelphia: W.B. Saunders Company; 1992.

Bolt, RJ; van Weissenbruch, MM; Lafeber, HN; Delemarre-van de Waal, HA. Glucocorticoids and lung development in the fetus and preterm infant. *Pediatr Pulmonol,* 2001, 32, 76-91.

Brand, PL; van Lingen, RA; Brus, F; Talsma, MD; Elzenga, NJ. Hypertrophic obstructive cardiomyopathy as a side effect of dexamethasone treatment for bronchopulmonary dysplasia. *Acta Paediatr,* 1993, 82, 614-617.

Brotman, DJ; Girod, JP; Garcia, MJ; Patel, JV; Gupta, M; Posch, A; Saunders, S; Lip, GY; Worley, S; Reddy, S. Effects of short-term glucocorticoids on cardiovascular biomarkers. *J Clin Endocrinol Metab,* 2005, 90, 3202-3208.

Burgess, AM; Hutchins GM. Inflammation of the lungs, umbilical cord and placenta associated with meconium passage in utero. Review of 123 autopsied cases. *Pathol Res Pract,* 1996, 192, 1121-1128.

Buttgereit, F; Brand, MD; Burmester, GR. Equivalent doses and relative drug potencies for non-genomic glucocorticoid effects: a novel glucocorticoid hierarchy. *Biochem Pharmacol* 1999, 58, 363-368.

Buttgereit, F. Mechanisms and clinical relevance of nongenomic glucocorticoid actions. *Z Rheumatol*, 2000, 59 Suppl 2:II, 119-123.

Buttgereit, F; Scheffold, A. Rapid glucocorticoid effects on immune cells. *Steroids*, 2002, 67, 529-534.

Cai, TQ; Wong, B; Mundt, SS; Thieringer, R; Wright, SD; Hermanowski-Vosatka, A. Induction of 11beta-hydroxysteroid dehydrogenase type 1 but not -2 in human aortic smooth muscle cells by inflammatory stimuli. *J Steroid Biochem Mol Biol*, 2001, 77, 117-122.

Castellheim, A; Lindenskov, PH; Pharo, A; Aamodt, G; Saugstad, OD; Mollness, TE. Meconium aspiration syndrome induces complement-associated systemic inflammatory response in newborn piglets. *Scand J Immunol,* 2005, 61, 217-225.

Chen, CM; Fang, CL; Chang, CH. Surfactant and corticosteroid effects on lung function in a rat model of acute lung injury. *Crit Care Med,* 2001, 29, 2169-2175.

Chen, YZ; Qiu, J. Possible genomic consequence of nongenomic action of glucocorticoids in neural cells. *News Physiol Sci,* 2001, 16, 292-296.

Co, E; Vidyasagar, D. Meconium aspiration syndrome. *Compr Ther,* 1990, 16, 34-39.

Craig, S; Lopez, A; Hoskin, D; Markham, F. Meconium inhibits phagocytosis and stimulates respiratory burst in alveolar macrophages. *Pediatr Res,* 2005, 57, 813-818.

Creuwels, LA; van Golde, LM; Haagsman, HP. The pulmonary surfactant system: biochemical and clinical aspects. *Lung,* 1997, 175, 1-39.

Crielaard, BJ; Lammers, T; Morgan, ME; Chaabane, L; Carboni, S; Greco, B; Zaratin, P; Kraneveld, AD; Storm, G. Macrophages and liposomes in inflammatory disease: friends or foes? *Int J Pharm,* 2011, 416, 499-506.

Cummings, DM; Larijani, GE; Conner, DP; Ferguson, RK; Rocci, ML Jr. Characterization of dexamethasone binding in normal and uremic human serum. *DICP,* 1990, 24, 229-231.

Czock, D; Keller, F; Rasche, FM; Häussler, U. Pharmacokinetics and pharmacodynamics of systemically administered glucocorticoids. *Clin Pharmacokinet,* 2005, 44, 61-98.

da Costa, DE; Nair, AK; Pai, MG; Al Khusaiby, SM. Steroids in full term infants with respiratory failure and pulmonary hypertension due to meconium aspiration syndrome. *Eur J Pediatr,* 2001, 160, 150-153.

Dargaville, PA. Respiratory support in meconium aspiration syndrome: a practical guide. *Int J Pediatr,* 2012a, 2012, 965159.

Dargaville, PA. Innovation in surfactant therapy I: surfactant lavage and surfactant administration by fluid bolus using minimally invasive techniques. *Neonatology,* 2012b, 101, 326-336.

Dargaville, PA; Copnell, B; Australian and New Zealand Neonatal Network. The epidemiology of meconium aspiration syndrome: Incidence, risk factors, therapies, and outcome. *Pediatrics,* 2006, 117, 1712-1721.

Dargaville, PA; Mills, JF. Surfactant therapy for meconium aspiration syndrome: current status. *Drugs,* 2005, 65, 2569-2591.

de Beaufort, AJ; Bakker, AC; van Tol, MJD; Poorthius, BJ; Schrama, AJ; Berger, HM. Meconium is a source of pro-inflammatory substances and can induce cytokine production in cultured A549 epithelial cells. *Pediatr Res,* 2003, 54, 491-495.

De Bosscher, K; Van Craenenbroeck, K; Meijer, OC; Haegeman, G. Selective transrepression versus transactivation mechanisms by glucocorticoid receptor modulators in stress and immune systems. *Eur J Pharmacol,* 2008, 583, 290-302.

De Bosscher, K. Selective Glucocorticoid Receptor modulators. *J Steroid Biochem Mol Biol,* 2010, 120, 96-104.

De Bosscher, K; Haegeman, G; Elewaut, D. Targeting inflammation using selective glucocorticoid receptor modulators. *Curr Opin Pharmacol,* 2010, 10, 497-504.

De Luca, D; Minucci, A; Tripodi, D; Piastra, M; Pietrini, D; Zuppi, C; Conti, G; Carnielli, VP; Capoluongo, E. Role of distinct phospholipases A2 and their modulators in meconium aspiration syndrome in human neonates. *Intensive Care Med,* 2011, 37, 1158-1165.

Diederich, S; Eigendorff, E; Burkhardt, P; Quinkler, M; Bumke-Vogt, C; Rochel, M; Seidelmann, D; Esperling, P; Oelkers, W; Bähr, V. 11beta-hydroxysteroid dehydrogenase types 1 and 2: an important pharmacokinetic determinant for the activity of synthetic mineralo- and glucocorticoids. *J Clin Endocrinol Metab*, 2002, 87, 5695-5701.

Diederich, S; Scholz, T; Eigendorff, E; Bumke-Vogt, C; Quinkler, M; Exner, P; Pfeiffer, AF; Oelkers, W; Bahr, V. Pharmacodynamics and pharmacokinetics of synthetic mineralocorticoids and glucocorticoids: receptor transactivation and prereceptor metabolism by 11beta-hydroxysteroid-dehydrogenases. *Horm Metabol Res,* 2004, 36, 423-429.

Diemel, RV; Snel, MM; Van Golde, LM; Putz, G; Haagsman, HP; Batenburg, JJ. Effects of cholesterol on surface activity and surface topography of spread surfactant films. *Biochemistry,* 2002, 41, 15007-15016.

Dubois, EFL. Clinical potencies of glucocorticoids: What do we really measure? *Curr Respir Med Rev,* 2005, 1, 103-108.

Durand, M; Mendoza, ME; Tantivit, P; Kugelman, A; McEvoy, C. A randomized trial of moderately early low-dose dexamethasone therapy in very low birth weight infants: dynamic pulmonary mechanics, oxygenation, and ventilation. *Pediatrics,* 2002, 109, 262-268.

Durham, PL; Wohlford-Lenane, CL; Snyder, JM. Glucocorticoid regulation of surfactant-associated proteins in rabbit fetal lung in vivo. *Anat Rec,* 1993, 237, 365-377.

Falkenstein, E; Tillmann, HC; Christ, M; Feuring, M; Wehling, M. Multiple actions of steroid hormones - a focus on rapid, nongenomic effects. *Pharmacol Rev*, 2000, 52, 513-556.

Fernandes, ABS; Zin, WA; Rocco, PRM. Corticosteroids in acute respiratory distress syndrome. *Braz J Med Biol Res,* 2005, 38, 147-159.

Fontanilla, R; Zagariya, A; Vidyasagar, D. Meconium-induced release of nitric oxide in rabbit alveolar cells. *J Perinatol,* 2008, 28 Suppl 3, S123-126.

Frantz, ID; Wang, NS; Thach, BT. Experimental meconium aspiration: Effects of glucocorticoid treatment. *J Pediatr,* 1975, 86, 438-441.

Frauman, AG. An overview of the adverse reactions to adrenal corticosteroids. *Adverse Drug React Toxicol Rev*, 1996, 15, 203-206.

Fuloria, M; Wiswell, TE. Resuscitation of the meconium-stained infant and prevention of meconium aspiration syndrome. *J Perinatol,* 1999, 19, 234-241.

Geiger, R; Kleinsasser, A; Meier, S; Neu, N; Pajk, W; Fischer, V; Treml, B; Stein, JI; Loeckinger, A. Intravenous tezosentan improves gas exchange and hemodynamics in acute lung injury secondary to meconium aspiration. *Intensive Care Med,* 2008, 34, 368-376.

Goldfarb, DS; Corbett, AH; Mason, DA; Harreman, MT; Adam, SA. Importin alpha: a multipurpose nuclear-transport receptor. *Trends Cell Biol,* 2004, 14, 505-514.

Goldsmith, JP. Continuous positive airway pressure and conventional mechanical ventilation in the treatment of meconium aspiration syndrome. *J Perinatol,* 2008, 28 Suppl 3, S49-S55.

Goulding, NJ. The molecular complexity of glucocorticoid actions in inflammation - a four-ring circus. *Curr Opin Pharmacol*, 2004, 4, 629-636.

Grier, DG; Halliday, HL. Effects of glucocorticoids on fetal and neonatal lung development. *Treat Respir Med,* 2004, 3, 295-306.

Gumprecht, K; Sieroń-Rokicka, B; Gumprecht, J; Grzeszczak, W. The influence of respiratory insufficiency on autonomic nervous system function in infants. *Wiad Lek,* 2002, 55, 373-381.

Halliday, HL. The effect of postnatal steroids on growth and development. *J Perinat Med*, 2001, 29, 281-285.

Hallman, M; Glumoff, V; Rämet, M. Surfactant in respiratory distress syndrome and lung injury. *Comp Biochem Physiol A Mol Integr Physiol,* 2001, 129, 287-294.

Holm, BA; Wang, Z; Notter, RH. Multiple mechanisms of lung surfactant inhibition. *Pediatr Res,* 1999, 46, 85-93.

Holopainen, R; Soukka, H; Halkola, L; Kääpä, P. Meconium aspiration induces a concentration-dependent pulmonary hypertensive response in newborn piglets. *Pediatr Pulmonol,* 1998, 25, 107-113.

Holopainen, R; Aho, H; Laine, J; Peuravuori, H; Soukka, H; Kääpä, P. Human meconium has high phospholipase A2 activity and induces cellular injury and apoptosis in piglet lungs. *Pediatr Res,* 1999, 46, 626-632.

Holopainen, R; Laine, J; Halkola, L; Aho, H; Kääpä, P. Dexamethasone treatment attenuates pulmonary injury in piglet meconium aspiration. *Pediatr Res,* 2001, 49, 162-168.

Isohama, Y; Rooney, SA. Glucocorticoid enhances the response of type II cells from newborn rats to surfactant secretagogues. *Biochim Biophys Acta,* 2001, 1531, 241-250.

Ito, K; Lim, S; Caramori, G; Chung, KF; Barnes, PJ; Adcock, IM. Cigarette smoking reduces histone deacetylase 2 expression, enhances cytokine expression, and inhibits glucocorticoid actions in alveolar macrophages. *FASEB J,* 2001, 15, 1110-1112.

Ito, K; Lim, S; Caramori, G; Cosio, B; Chung, KF; Adcock, IM; Barnes, PJ. A molecular mechanism of action of theophylline: induction of histone deacetylase activity to decrease inflammatory gene expression. *Proc Natl Acad Sci USA,* 2002, 99, 8921-8926.

Jantz, MA; Sahn, AS. Corticosteroids in acute respiratory failure. *Am J Respir Crit Care Med,* 1999, 160, 1079-1100.

Jeng, MJ; Soong, WJ; Lee, YS; Chang, HL; Shen, CM; Wang, CH; Yang, SS; Hwang, B. Effects of therapeutic bronchoalveolar lavage and partial liquid ventilation on meconium-aspirated newborn piglets. *Crit Care Med,* 2006, 34, 1099-1105.

Jones, RA. Collaborative Dexamethasone Trial Follow-up Group. Randomized, controlled trial of dexamethasone in neonatal chronic lung disease: 13- to 17-year follow-up study: II. Respiratory status, growth, and blood pressure. *Pediatrics,* 2005, 116, 379-384.

Kääpä, PO. Meconium aspiration syndrome (MAS) - Where do we go? Research perspectives. *Early Hum Dev,* 2009, 85, 627-629.

Katz, VL; Bowes, WA Jr. Meconium aspiration syndrome: reflections on a murky subject. *Am J Obstet Gynecol,* 1992, 166, 171-183.

Katzung, BG; Masters, SB; Trevor AJ, eds. *Basic and Clinical Pharmacology.* 12th ed. New York, NY: McGraw-Hill Lange, 2012, 1248.

Kawai, S; Ichikawa, Y; Homma, M. Differences in metabolic properties among cortisol, prednisolone, and dexamethasone in liver and renal diseases: accelerated metabolism of dexamethasone in renal failure. *J Clin Endocrinol Metab,* 1985, 60, 848-854.

Khan, AM; Shabarek, FM; Kutchback, JW; Lally, KP. Effects of dexamethasone on meconium aspiration syndrome in newborn piglets. *Pediatr Res,* 1999, 46, 179-183.

Khan, AM; Elidemir, O; Epstein, CE; Lally, KP; Xue, H; Blackburn, M; Larsen, GL; Colasurdo, GN. Meconium aspiration produces airway hyperresponsiveness and eosinophilic inflammation in murine model. *Am J Physiol Lung Cell Mol Physiol,* 2002a, 283, L785-L790.

Khan, AM; Lally, KP; Elidemir, O; Colasurdo, GN. Meconium enhances the release of nitric oxide in human airway epithelial cells. *Biol Neonate,* 2002b, 81, 99-104.

Khan, AM; Lally, KP; Larsen, GL; Colasurdo, GN. Enhanced release of thromboxane A(2) after exposure of human airway epithelial cells to meconium. *Pediatr Pulmonol,* 2002c, 33, 111-116.

Kirimi, E; Tuncer, O; Kosem, M; Ceylan, E; Tas, A; Tasal, I; Balahoroglu, R; Caksen, H. The effects of prednisolone and serum malondialdehyde levels in puppies with experimentally induced meconium aspiration syndrome. *J Int Med Res,* 2003, 31, 113-122.

Klingner, MC; Kruse, J. Meconium aspiration syndrome: pathophysiology and prevention. *J Am Board Fam Pract,* 1999, 12, 450-466.

Koukouritaki, SB; Theodoropoulos, PA; Margioris, AN; Gravanis, A; Stournaras, C. Dexamethasone alters rapidly actin polymerization dynamics in human endometrial cells: evidence for nongenomic actions involving cAMP turnover. *J Cell Biochem,* 1996, 62, 251-261.

Kuo, CY; Chen, JY. Effects of meconium aspiration on plasma endothelin-1 level and pulmonary hemodynamics in a piglet model. *Biol Neonate,* 1999, 76, 228-234.

Kytola, J; Kääpä, P; Uotila, P. Meconium aspiration stimulates cyclooxygenase-2 and nitric oxide synthase-2 expression in rat lungs. *Pediatr Res,* 2003, 53, 731-736.

Larsson, M; Nylander, T; Keough, KM; Nag, K. An X-ray diffraction study of alterations in bovine lung surfactant bilayer structures induced by albumin. *Chem Phys Lipids,* 2006, 144, 137-145.

Le Cras, TD; Markham, NE; Morris, KG; Ahrens, CR; McMurtry, IF; Abman, SH. Neonatal dexamethasone treatment increases the risk for pulmonary hypertension in adult rats. *Am J Physiol Lung Cell Mol Physiol,* 2000, 278, L822-L829.

Lee, SR; Kim, HK; Youm, JB; Dizon, LA; Song, IS; Jeong, SH; Seo, DY; Ko, KS; Rhee, BD; Kim, N; Han, J. Non-genomic effect of glucocorticoids on cardiovascular system. *Pflugers Arch,* 2012, 464, 549-559.

Lewis, GP; Jusko, WJ; Graves, L; Burke, CW. Prednisone side-effects and serum-protein levels: a collaborative study. *Lancet,* 1971, II(7728), 778-780.

Li, YH; Yan, ZQ; Brauner, A; Tullus, K. Meconium induces expression of inducible NO synthase and activation of NF-kappaB in rat alveolar macrophages. *Pediatr Res,* 2001, 49, 820-825.

Lifton, RP; Gharavi, AG; Geller, DS. Molecular mechanisms of human hypertension. *Cell,* 2001, 104, 545-556.

Liu, L; Wang, YX; Zhou, J; Long, F; Sun, HW; Liu, Y; Chen, YZ; Jiang, CL. Rapid non-genomic inhibitory effects of glucocorticoids on human neutrophil degranulation. *Inflamm Res,* 2005, 54, 37-41.

Long, F; Wang, YX; Liu, L; Zhou, J; Cui, RY; Jiang, CL. Rapid nongenomic inhibitory effects of glucocorticoids on phagocytosis and superoxide anion production by macrophages. *Steroids*, 2005, 70, 55-61.

Lopez-Rodriguez, E; Echaide, M; Cruz, A; Taeusch, HW; Perez-Gil, J. Meconium impairs pulmonary surfactant by a combined action of cholesterol and bile acids. *Biophys J,* 2011, 100, 646-655.

Lösel, R; Wehling, M. Nongenomic actions of steroid hormones. *Nat Rev Mol Cell Biol*, 2003, 4, 46-56.

Löwenberg, M; Verhaar, AP; van den Brink, GR; Hommes, DW. Glucocorticoid signaling: a nongenomic mechanism for T-cell immunosuppression. *Trends Mol Med,* 2007, 13, 158-163.

Löwenberg, M; Stahn, C; Hommes, DW; Buttgereit, F. Novel insights into mechanisms of glucocorticoid action and the development of new glucocorticoid receptor ligands. *Steroids,* 2008, 73, 1025-1029.

Mager, DE; Jusko, WJ. Quantitative structure-pharmacokinetic/ pharmacodynamic relationships of corticosteroids in man. *J Pharm Sci*, 2002, 91, 2441-2451.

Markham, A; Faulds, D. Theophylline: a review of its potential steroid sparing effects in asthma. *Drugs*, 1998, 56, 1081-1091.

Marsland, AL; Gianaros, PJ; Prather, AA; Jennings, JR; Neumann, SA; Manuck, SB. Stimulated production of proinflammatory cytokines covaries inversely with heart rate variability. *Psychosom Med,* 2007, 69, 709-716.

McColl, A; Michlewska, S; Dransfield, I; Rossi, AG. Effects of glucocorticoids on apoptosis and clearance of apoptotic cells. *Scientific World Journal*, 2007, 7, 1165-1181.

Merz, U; Kusenbach, G; Häusler, M; Peschgens, T; Hörnchen, H. Inhaled budesonide in ventilator-dependent preterm infants: a randomized, double-blind pilot study. *Biol Neonate,* 1999, 75, 46-53.

Moguilevski, VA; Shiel, L; Oliver, J; McGrath, BP. Power spectral analysis of heart-rate variability reflects the level of cardiac autonomic activity in rabbits. *J Auton Nerv Syst,* 1996, 58, 18-24.

Mokra, D; Calkovska, A; Tonhajzerova, I; Petraskova, M; Bulikova, J; Redfors, B; Javorka, K. Intratracheal budesonide improved the lung functions in meconium-instilled rabbits without side effects on cardiovascular functions. *Eur Respir J*, 2007a, 30 Suppl 51, 396p.

Mokra, D; Mokry, J; Drgova, A; Petraskova, M; Bulikova, J, Calkovska, A. Intratracheally administered corticosteroids improve lung function in meconium-instilled rabbits. *J Physiol Pharmacol,* 2007b, 58 (Suppl 5), 389-398.

Mokra, D; Mokry, J; Drgova, A; Bulikova, J; Petraskova, M; Calkovska, A. Single-dose vs. two-dose dexamethasone effects on lung inflammation and airway reactivity in meconium-instilled rabbits. *J Physiol Pharmacol,* 2007c, 58 (Suppl 5), 379-387.

Mokra, D; Calkovska, A; Tonhajzerova, I; Petraskova, M; Bulikova, J; Redfors, B. Dexamethasone treatment improved lung functions in meconium-instilled rabbits, but influenced cardiovascular variables. *Bratisl Med J*, 2008a, 109, 95-101.

Mokra, D; Drgova, A; Mokry, J; Bulikova, J; Pullmann, R; Durdik, P; Petraskova, M; Calkovska, A. Combination of budesonide and aminophylline diminished acute lung injury in animal model of meconium aspiration syndrome. *J Physiol Pharmacol*, 2008b, 59 Suppl 6, 461-471.

Mokra, D; Tonhajzerova, I; Mokry, J; Drgova, A; Petraskova, M; Calkovska, A; Javorka, K. Rapid cardiovascular effects of dexamethasone in rabbits with meconium-induced acute lung injury. *Can J Physiol Pharmacol*, 2008c, 86, 804-814.

Mokra, D; Tonhajzerova, I; Petraskova, M; Calkovska, A. Effects of dexamethasone on cardiovascular functions in acute phase in meconium-injured rabbits. *Pediatr Int,* 2009, 51, 132-137.

Mokra, D; Mokry, J. Meconium aspiration syndrome. From pathomechanisms to treatment. 1st Edition. New York: Nova Science Publishers; 2010.

Mokra, D; Mokry, J. Glucocorticoids in the treatment of neonatal meconium aspiration syndrome. *Eur J Pediatr,* 2011, 170, 1495-1505.

Mokry, J; Mokra, D; Antosova, M; Bulikova, J; Calkovska, A; Nosalova, G. Dexamethasone alleviates meconium-induced airway hyperresponsiveness and lung inflammation in rabbits. *Pediatr Pulmonol,* 2006, 41, 55-60.

Murray, DR. What is "heart rate variability" and is it blunted by tumor necrosis factor? *Chest,* 2003, 123, 664-667.

Muto, S; Ebata, S; Okada, K; Saito, T; Asano, Y. Glucocorticoid modulates Na+/H+ exchange activity in vascular smooth muscle cells by nongenomic and genomic mechanisms. *Kidney Int,* 2000, 57, 2319-2333.

Newton, R. Molecular mechanisms of glucocorticoid action: what is important? *Thorax,* 2000, 55, 603-613.

Nimmo, AJ; Carstairs, JR; Patole, SK; Whitehall, J; Davidson, K; Vink, R. Intratracheal administration of glucocorticoids using surfactant as a vehicle. *Clin Exp Pharmacol Physiol,* 2002, 29, 661-665.

Nupponen, I; Repo, H; Kari, A; Pohjavuori, M; Andersson, S. Early dexamethasone decreases expression of activation markers on neutrophils and monocytes in preterm infants. *Acta Paediatr*, 2002, 91, 1200-1207.

Okajima, S; Matsuda, T; Cho, K; Matsumoto, Y; Kobayashi, Y; Fujimoto, S. Antenatal dexamethasone administration impairs normal postnatal lung growth in rats. *Pediatr Res,* 2001, 49, 777-781.

Paul-Clark, MJ; Roviezzo, F; Flower, RJ; Cirino, G; Soldato, PD; Adcock, IM; Perretti, M. Glucocorticoid receptor nitration leads to enhanced anti-inflammatory effects of novel steroid ligands. *J Immunol,* 2003, 171, 3245-3252.

Perretti, M; Paul-Clark, MJ; Mancini, L; Flower, RJ. Generation of innovative anti-inflammatory and anti-arthritic glucocorticoid derivatives that release NO: the nitro-steroids. *Dig Liver Dis,* 2003, 35 Suppl 2, S41-S48.

Pratt, WB; Galigniana, MD; Harrell, JM; DeFranco, DB. Role of hsp90 and the hsp90-binding immunophilins in signalling protein movement. *Cell Signal,* 2004, 16, 857-872.

Price, LC; Montani, D; Tcherakian, C; Dorfmüller, P; Souza, R; Gambaryan, N; Chaumais, M-C; Shao, DM; Simonneau, G; Howard, LS; Adcock, IM; Wort, SJ; Humbert, M; Perros, F. Dexamethasone reverses monocrotaline-induced pulmonary arterial hypertension in rats. *Eur Respir J,* 2011, 37, 813-822.

Ramin, SM; Vidaeff, AC; Gilstrap, LC 3rd; Bishop, KD; Jenkins, GN; Alcorn, JL. The effects of dexamethasone and betamethasone on surfactant protein-B messenger RNA expression in human type II pneumocytes and human lung adenocarcinoma cells. *Am J Obstet Gynecol,* 2004, 190, 952-959.

Rastogi, A; Akintorin, SM; Bez, ML; Morales, P; Pildes, RS. A controlled trial of dexamethasone to prevent bronchopulmonary dysplasia in surfactant-treated infants. *Pediatrics,* 1996, 98, 204-210.

Rey-Santano, C; Mielgo, VE; Gastiasoro, E; Alvarez-Diaz, FJ; Lafuente, H; Valls-i-Soler, A; Murgia, X. Comparative effects of bronchoalveolar lavage with saline, surfactant, or perfluorocarbon in experimental meconium aspiration syndrome. *Pediatr Crit Care Med,* 2012, 13, e187-e194

Rhen, T; Cidlowski, JA. Antiinflammatory action of glucocorticoids--new mechanisms for old drugs. *N Engl J Med,* 2005, 353, 1711-1723.

Rodríguez-Capote, K; Manzanares, D; Haines, T; Possmayer, F. Reactive oxygen species inactivation of surfactant involves structural and functional alterations to surfactant proteins SP-B and SP-C. *Biophys J,* 2006, 90, 2808-2821.

Rohdewald, P; Möllmann, H; Barth, J; Rehder, J; Derendorf, H. Pharmacokinetics of dexamethasone and its phosphate ester. *Biopharm Drug Dispos,* 1987, 8, 205-212.

Rose, JQ; Yurchak, AM; Jusko, WJ. Dose dependent pharmacokinetics of prednisone and prednisolone in man. *J Pharmacokinet Biopharm*, 1981, 9, 389-417.

Rosman, PM; Benn, R; Kay, M; Tito, J; Wallace, EZ. Cortisol binding in uremic plasma. I: Absence of abnormal cortisol binding to cortisol binding to corticosteroid-binding globulin. *Nephron*, 1984, 37, 160-165.

Roth, M; Johnson, PR; Rüdiger, JJ; King, GG; Ge, Q; Burgess, JK; Anderson, G; Tamm, M; Black, JL. Interaction between glucocorticoids and β2 agonists on bronchial airway smooth muscle cells through synchronised cellular signalling. *Lancet*, 2002, 360, 1293-1299.

Sáenz, A; López-Sánchez, A; Mojica-Lázaro, J; Martínez-Caro, L; Nin, N; Bagatolli, LA; Casals, C. Fluidizing effects of C-reactive protein on lung surfactant membranes: protective role of surfactant protein A. *FASEB J,* 2010, 24, 3662-3673.

Salvia-Roiges, MD; Carbonell-Estrany, X; Figueras-Aloy, J; Rodriguez-Miquelez, JM. Efficacy of three treatment schedules in severe meconium aspiration syndrome. *Acta Paediatr,* 2004, 93, 60-65.

Sanders, RJ; Cox, C; Phelps, DL; Sinkin, RA. Two doses of early intravenous dexamethasone for the prevention of bronchopulmonary dysplasia in babies with respiratory distress syndrome. *Pediatr Res,* 1994, 36, 122-128.

Schäcke, H; Döcke, WD; Asadullah, K. Mechanisms involved in the side effects of glucocorticoids. *Pharmacology & Therapeutics,* 2002, 96, 23-43.

Scheuer, DA; Bechtold, AG. Glucocorticoids potentiate central actions of angiotensin to increase arterial pressure. *Am J Physiol Regul Integr Comp Physiol,* 2001, 280, R1719-R1726.

Scheuer, DA; Mifflin, SW. Glucocorticoids modulate baroreflex control of renal sympathetic nerve activity. *Am J Physiol Regul Integr Comp Physiol,* 2001, 280, R1440-R1449.

Schmid, D; Burmester, GR; Tripmacher, R; Kuhnke, A; Buttgereit, F. Bioenergetics of human peripheral blood mononuclear cell metabolism in quiescent, activated, and glucocorticoid-treated states. *Biosci Rep,* 2000, 20, 289-302.

Schrama, AJ; de Beaufort, AJ; Sukul, YR; Jansen, SM; Poorthuis, BJ; Berger, HM. Phospholipase A2 is present in meconium and inhibits the activity of pulmonary surfactant: an in vitro study. *Acta Paediatr,* 2001, 90, 412-416.

Schweingruber, N; Haine, A; Tiede, K; Karabinskaya, A; van den Brandt, J; Wüst, S; Metselaar, JM; Gold, R; Tuckermann, JP; Reichardt, HM; Lühder, F. Liposomal encapsulation of glucocorticoids alters their mode of action in the treatment of experimental autoimmune encephalomyelitis. *J Immunol,* 2011, 187, 4310-4318.

Shi, WL; Ma, Q; Zhang, LD; Huang, JL; Zhou, J; Liu, L; Shen, XH; Jiang, CL. Corticosterone rapidly promotes respiratory burst of mouse peritoneal macrophages via non-genomic mechanism. *Chin Med J (Engl),* 2011, 124, 3127-3132.

Shinwell, ES; Karplus, M; Reich, D; Weintraub, Z; Blazer, S; Bader, D; Yurman, S; Dolfin, T; Kogan, A; Dollberg, S; Arbel, E; Goldberg, M; Gur, I; Naor, N; Sirota, L; Mogilner, S; Zaritsky, A; Barak, M; Gottfried, E. Early postnatal dexamethasone treatment and increased incidence of cerebral palsy. *Arch Dis Child Fetal Neonatal Ed,* 2000, 83, F177-F181.

Silvera, FE; Blasina, MF; Vaamonde, L; Tellechea, S; Godoy, C; Zabala, S; Mañana, G; Martell, M; Olivera, W. Sildenafil prevents the increase of extravascular lung water and pulmonary hypertension after meconium aspiration in newborn piglets. *Braz J Med Biol Res,* 2011, 44, 778-85.

Skelton, R; Gill, AB; Parsons, JM. Cardiac effects of short course dexamethasone in preterm infants. *Arch Dis Child Fetal Neonatal Ed,* 1998, 78, F133-F137.

Soukka, H; Halkola, L; Aho, H; Rautanen, M; Kero, P; Kääpä, P. Methylprednisolone attenuates the pulmonary hypertensive response in porcine meconium aspiration. *Pediatr Res,* 1997, 42, 145-150.

Soukka, H; Viinika, L; Kääpä, P. Involvement of thromboxane A_2 and prostacyclin in the early pulmonary hypertension after porcine meconium aspiration. *Pediatr Res,* 1998, 44, 838-842.

Soukka, HR; Ahotupa, M; Ruutu, M; Kääpä, PO. Meconium stimulates neutrophil oxidative burst. *Am J Perinatol,* 2002, 19, 279-284.

Stahn, C; Löwenberg, M; Hommes, DW; Buttgereit, F. Molecular mechanisms of glucocorticoid action and selective glucocorticoid receptor agonists. *Mol Cell Endocrinol,* 2007, 275, 71-78.

Stark, AR; Carlo, WA; Tyson, JE; Papile, LA; Wright, LL; Shankaran, S; Donovan, EF; Oh, W; Bauer, CR; Saha, S; Poole, WK; Stoll, BJ; National Institute of Child Health and Human Development Neonatal Research Network. Adverse effects of early dexamethasone in extremely-low-birth-weight infants. National Institute of Child Health and Human Development Neonatal Research Network. *N Engl J Med*, 2001, 344, 95-101.

Steinhorn, RH. Nitric oxide and beyond: new insights and therapies for pulmonary hypertension. *J Perinatol,* 2008, 28 Suppl 3, S67-S71.

Stellato, C. Post-transcriptional and nongenomic effects of glucocorticoids. *Proc Am Thorac Soc*, 2004, 1, 255-263.

Suchomski, SJ; Cummings, JJ. A randomized trial of inhaled versus intravenous steroids in ventilator-dependent preterm infants. *J Perinatol,* 2002, 22, 196-203.

Sun, HW; Miao, CY; Liu, L; Zhou, J; Su, DF; Wang, YX; Jiang, CL. Rapid inhibitory effect of glucocorticoids on airway smooth muscle contractions in guinea pigs. *Steroids,* 2006, 71, 154-159.

Tao, T; Lan, J; Lukacs, GL; Haché, RJ; Kaplan, F. Importin 13 regulates nuclear import of the glucocorticoid receptor in airway epithelial cells. *Am J Respir Cell Mol Biol,* 2006, 35, 668-680.

Tapia, JL; Ramírez, R; Cifuentes, J; Fabres, J; Hübner, ME; Bancalari, A; Mercado, ME; Standen, J; Escobar, M. The effect of early dexamethasone administration on bronchopulmonary dysplasia in preterm infants with respiratory distress syndrome. *J Pediatr,* 1998, 132, 48-52.

Thieringer, R; Le Grand, CB; Carbin, L; Cai, TQ; Wong, B; Wright, SD; Hermanowski-Vosatka, A. 11 Beta-hydroxysteroid dehydrogenase type 1 is induced in human monocytes upon differentiation to macrophages. *J Immunol,* 2001, 167, 30-35.

Thureen, PJ; Hall, DM; Hoffenberg, A; Tyson, RW. Fatal meconium aspiration in spite of appropriate perinatal airway management: Pulmonary and placental evidence of prenatal disease. *Am J Obstet Gynecol,* 1997, 176, 1-9.

Tingay, DG; Mills, JF; Morley, CJ; Pellicano, A; Dargaville, PA; Australian and New Zealand Neonatal Network. Trends in use and outcome of newborn infants treated with high frequency ventilation in Australia and New Zealand, 1996-2003. *J Paediatr Child Health,* 2007, 43, 160-166.

Tomlinson, JW; Walker, EA; Bujalska, I; Draper, N; Lavery, GG; Cooper, MS; Hewison, M; Stewart, PM. 11β-Hydroxysteroid dehydrogenase type 1: a tissue-specific regulator of glucocorticoid response. *Endocr Rev* 2004, 25, 831-866.

Tran, N; Lowe, C; Sivieri, EM; Shaffer, TH. Sequential effects of acute meconium obstruction on pulmonary function. *Pediatr Res,* 1980, 14, 34-38.

Tripathi, S; Saili, A. The effect of steroids on the clinical course and outcome of neonates with meconium aspiration syndrome. *J Trop Pediatr,* 2007, 53, 8-12.

Tripathi, S; Saili, A; Dutta, R. Inflammatory markers in meconium induced lung injury in neonates and effect of steroids on their levels: a randomized controlled trial. *Indian J Med Microbiol,* 2007, 25, 103-107.

Türüt, H; Ciralik, H; Kilinc, M; Ozbag, D; Imrek, SS. Effects of early administration of dexamethasone, N-acetylcysteine and aprotinin on inflammatory and oxidant-antioxidant status after lung contusion in rats. *Injury,* 2009, 40, 521-527.

Tyler, DC; Murphy, J; Cheney, FW. Mechanical and chemical damage to lung tissue caused by meconium aspiration. *Pediatrics,* 1978, 62, 454-459.

Ullian, ME. The role of corticosteroids in the regulation of vascular tone. *Cardiovasc Res,* 1999, 41, 55-64.

Uotila, PJ; Kääpä, PO. Cyclooxygenase-2 expression in human monocytes stimulated by meconium. *Lancet,* 1998, 351, 878.

Urbach, V; Walsh, DE; Mainprice, B; Bousquet, J; Harvey, BJ. Rapid non-genomic inhibition of ATP-induced Cl- secretion by dexamethasone in human bronchial epithelium. *J Physiol,* 2002, 545, 869-878.

van den Anker, JN; van Loenen, NTVM. Dexamethasone in meconium aspiration. *Eur J Pediatr,* 1994, 153, 864.

van Ierland, Y; de Beaufort, AJ. Why does meconium cause meconium aspiration syndrome? Current concepts of MAS pathophysiology. *Early Hum Dev*, 2009, 85, 617-620.

Vázquez Nava, F; Salas Ramírez, E; Sánchez Núncio, HR; Saldivar González, AH; Beltrán Saldaňa, J; Cadena Mata, D; Pérez Rodríguez, P; Pérez Martin, J; Almeida, VM; Guidos Fogelbach, G. Meconium aspiration syndrome, parental atopy and asthma symptoms in children under two years old. *Rev Alerg Mex,* 2006, 53, 130-135.

Verriére, VA; Hynes, D; Faherty, S; Devaney, J; Bousquet, J; Harvey, BJ; Urbach, V. Rapid effects of dexamethasone on intracellular pH and Na^+/H^+ exchanger activity in human bronchial epithelial cells. *J Biol Chem,* 2005, 280, 35807-35814.

Vidyasagar, D; Lukkarinen, H; Kaapa, P; Zagariya, A. Inflammatory response and apoptosis in newborn lungs after meconium aspiration. *Biotechnol Prog,* 2005, 21, 192-197.

Vidyasagar, D; Zagariya, A. Studies of meconium-induced lung injury: inflammatory cytokine expression and apoptosis. *J Perinatol,* 2008, 28 Suppl 3, S102-S107.

Walker, BR. Extra-adrenal regeneration of glucocorticoids by 11beta-hydroxysteroid dehydrogenase type 1: physiological regulator and pharmacological target for energy partitioning. *Proc Nutr Soc,* 2007a, 66, 1-8.

Walker, BR. Glucocorticoids and cardiovascular disease. *Eur J Endocrinol,* 2007b, 157, 545-559.

Wang, JY; Yeh, TF; Lin, YJ; Chen, WY; Lin, CH. Early postnatal dexamethasone therapy may lessen lung inflammation in premature infants with respiratory distress syndrome on mechanical ventilation. *Pediatr Pulmonol,* 1997, 23, 193-197.

Wehling, M. Specific nongenomic actions of steroid hormones. *Ann Rev Physiol,* 1997, 59, 365-393.

Wiedmann, TS; Bhatia, R; Wattenberg, LW. Drug solubilization in lung surfactant. *J Control Release,* 2000, 65, 43-47.

Wiswell, TE; Bent, RC. Meconium staining and the meconium aspiration syndrome. Unresolved issues. *Pediatr Clin North Am,* 1993, 40, 955-981.

Wu, JM; Yeh, TF; Wang, JY; Lin, YJ; Hsieh, WS; Lin, CH. The role of pulmonary inflammation in the development of pulmonary hypertension in newborn with meconium aspiration syndrome (MAS). *Pediatr Pulmonol,* 1999, Suppl 18, 205-208.

Yamada, T; Minakami, H; Matsubara, S; Yatsuda, T; Kohmura, Y; Sato, I. Meconium-stained amniotic fluid exhibits chemotactic activity for polymorphonuclear leukocytes in vitro. *J Reprod Immunol,* 2000, 46, 21-30.

Yeh, TF; Lin, YJ; Hsieh, WS; Lin, HC; Lin, CH; Chen, JY; Kao, HA; Chien, CH. Early postnatal dexamethasone therapy for the prevention of chronic lung disease in preterm infants with respiratory distress syndrome: a multicenter clinical trial. *Pediatrics,* 1997, 100, E3.

Yeh, TF; Lin, YJ; Huang, CC; Chen, YJ; Lin, CH; Lin, HC; Hsieh, WS; Lien, YJ. Early dexamethasone therapy in preterm infants: a follow-up study. *Pediatrics,* 1998, 101, E7.

Yeh, TF; Srinivasan, G; Harris, V; Pildes, RS. Hydrocortisone therapy in meconium aspiration syndrome: a controlled study. *J Pediatr,* 1977, 90, 140-143.

Zagariya, A; Bhat, R; Chari, G; Uhal, B; Navale, S; Vidyasagar, D. Apoptosis of airway epithelial cells in response to meconium. *Life Sci,* 2005, 76, 1849-1858.

Zagariya, A; Bhat, R; Navale, S; Chari, G; Vidyasagar, D. Inhibition of meconium-induced cytokine expression and cell apoptosis by pretreatment with captopril. *Pediatrics,* 2006, 117, 1722-1727.

Zagariya, A; Bhat, R; Navale, S; Vidyasagar, D. Cytokine expression in meconium-induced lungs. *Indian J Pediatr,* 2004, 71, 195-201.

Zhou, J; Kang, ZM; Xie, QM; Liu, C; Lou, SJ; Chen, YZ; Jiang, CL. Rapid nongenomic effects of glucocorticoids on allergic asthma reaction in the guinea pig. *J Endocrinol,* 2003, 177, R1-R4.

Zuo, YY; Veldhuize, RA; Neumann, AW; Petersen, NO; Possmayer, F. Current perspectives in pulmonary surfactant - Inhibition, enhancement and evaluation. *Biochim Biophys Acta,* 2008, 1778, 1947-1977.

Reviewed by:

Anna Drgova, RND., PhD., Assoc. Prof., Department of Biochemistry, Jessenius Faculty of Medicine, Comenius University, Martin, Slovakia;

Anna Strapkova, RND., PhD., Assoc. Prof., Department of Pharmacology, Jessenius Faculty of Medicine, Comenius University, Martin, Slovakia.

In: Dexamethasone
Editors: A. Sauvage and M. Levy
ISBN: 978-1-62808-405-4

Chapter II

Dexamethasone Effects in Hyperinfection Syndrome due to Strongyloidiasis

***Cristiane Tefé-Silva*[1]*, Daniela I. Souza*[2]*, Eleuza R. Machado*[2,3]*, Karina M. Mata*[1]*, Margaret de Castro*[4]*, Lúcia H. Faccioli*[2] *and Simone G. Ramos*[1*]**

[1] Department of Pathology, Faculty of Medicine of Ribeirão Preto, University of São Paulo, São Paulo, Brazil
[2] Department of Clinical Analyses, Toxicology and Bromatology, School of Pharmaceutical Sciences of Ribeirão Preto, University of São Paulo, Ribeirão Preto, Brazil
[3] Brasília Anhanguera Faculty, Brasília, Brazil
[4] Department of Medical Clinic, School of Medicine of Ribeirão Preto, University of São Paulo, Ribeirão Preto, Brazil

[*] E-mail address: sgramos@fmrp.usp.br.

Abstract

Background: Dexamethasone is a synthetic corticosteroid with anti-inflammatory effects that is widely used to treat autoimmune and other chronic inflammatory diseases. Prolonged treatment with dexamethasone can result in the development of hyperinfection syndrome in strongyloidiasis through several different mechanisms. This complication can be relevant in areas where *Strongyloides* species are endemic, rendering hyperinfection syndrome an important global health problem.

Material and Methods: Rats inoculated with 9 x 10^3 *Strongyloides venezuelensis* larvae and treated with dexamethasone were sacrificed on days 1, 3, 5, 7, 14 and 21. The lungs, spleen, kidney, heart, liver, and brain were harvested, minced and incubated, so that migrating larvae could be collected and counted under a light microscope. Eosinophils and mononuclear cells were quantified from blood samples, BALF (bronchoalveolar lavage fluid) and PCF (peritoneal cavity fluid). Interleukin levels were evaluated using an ELISA assay. Corticosterone and ecdysteroid were measured in parasite cultures. Glucocorticoid receptor protein levels were assessed in parasite extracts by Western immunoblot analysis.

Results: Dexamethasone-treated rats carried increased parasite burdens and had enhanced female worm fertility, which induced steroid-hormone overproduction by the parasites, likely via an increase in the synthesis of corticosterone and ecdysone-like hormones. Dexamethasone also reduced eosinophil and mononuclear cell numbers and inhibited interleukins such as IL-1β and IL-4, culminating with the dissemination of larvae to other organs indicating a progression toward hyperinfection and death.

Conclusion: Dexamethasone decreases the Th2-type immune response to parasitic infection, ultimately leading to septic shock and the dissemination of larvae to other organs. Furthermore, dexamethasone may play a direct role in promoting worm proliferation. Further experimental studies are essential to elucidate the parasite's behavior and the role of the immune system in strongyloidiasis, particularly in patients using dexamethasone to treat hyperinfection syndrome. These studies contribute to the understanding of the molecular basis of infection and help to prevent hyperinfection syndrome in strongyloidiasis, which has a high mortality rate.

Keywords: Glucocorticoids, dexamethasone, hyperinfection syndrome, strongyloidiasis

1. Introduction

Strongyloides species are nematode parasites estimated to infect approximately 100 million people worldwide. They are generally found in warm, moist areas due to the suitability of such climates for survival at the larval stage [1, 2]. The worm has a complex life cycle in humans and other animals. Infections are initiated by larval penetration of the skin, and these larvae subsequently travel through the bloodstream to the lungs, where they migrate into the alveolar spaces, ascend the respiratory tree, and are swallowed. The larvae then continue their development in the small intestine [3].

Most infected individuals are asymptomatic; however, other individuals can present with a variety of symptoms, such as coughing, shortness of breath, wheezing and transient pulmonary infiltrates. Although the majority of these infections are resolved [4], a peculiar aspect of *Strongyloides* parasitosis, termed autoinfection, has been described [3, 5]. Autoinfection refers to the process by which larvae can re-infect the host by invading the intestinal wall, persisting indefinitely in the infected hosts [3, 6, 7]. Moreover, in immunocompromised hosts, autoinfection can lead to an accelerated hyperinfective cycle, resulting in a massive larval invasion that can potentially lead to a life-threatening illness with multi-organ failure and death as the outcome [8, 9, 10]. This syndrome, commonly referred to as hyperinfection syndrome, occurs most often in patients receiving corticosteroids [11, 12]. In addition to modulating host immunity, corticosteroids appear to interact with the steroid metabolism of parasite larvae themselves, leading to an increased worm burden and thus favoring dissemination of infection [13].

2. Glucocorticoids

Corticosteroids are highly effective anti-inflammatory drugs used to treat inflammatory and autoimmune diseases. They produce potent effects by inducing or repressing the expression of target genes [14]. Protein, carbohydrate and lipid metabolism, as well as electrolyte levels, are all regulated by corticosteroids [15].

Corticosteroids exert their effects utilizing three classes of hormones synthesized in different subregions of the adrenal cortex: the zona glumerulosa (mineralocorticoids), the zona fasciculata (glucocorticoids) and the zona reticulata (androgens) [16]. Glucocorticoids (GCs) are essential for the metabolism of carbohydrates, proteins and lipids, the regulation of circadian rhythms, the regulation of the reproductive system, and the activation of the immune response; thus, glucocorticoids are crucial for human survival in that they exert their effects on all tissues and organs. In addition, glucocorticoids activate and suppress many pro- and anti-inflammatory genes and exert post-transcriptional effects [17].

2.1. Metabolism

The hypothalamus-pituitary adrenal (HPA) axis increases corticotrophin releasing hormone (CRH), which leads to the synthesis of adrenocorticotropic hormone (ACTH). ACTH then stimulates the adrenal cortex, resulting in adrenal hyperplasia and the production of GCs [18, 15]. The HPA axis induces the secretion of glucocorticoids (human cortisol or rodent corticosterone) from the adrenal cortex [19].

2.2. Mechanism of Action

Both endogenous (cortisol in humans) and synthetic (dexamethasone, prednisolone) GCs are lipophilic; thus, they enter cells by diffusing across cell membranes and binding to glucocorticoid receptors (GRs) in the cytoplasm. The GR gene is located on chromosome 5q31-32 and contains nine exons, which are widely preserved across species [18].

GRs are activated by proteins and released from molecular chaperones such as heat shock protein-90 (hsp-90). Activated GRs translocate into the nucleus, where they bind to DNA at GREs (glucocorticoid response elements), which are specific sequences in the promoter region of corticosteroid-response genes [14]. The interaction of an activated GR dimer with a GRE results in the suppression of pro-inflammatory genes through direct binding of the GR to GREs [18, 20]. Numerous genes that are switched on by corticosteroids exert anti-inflammatory effects and may increase the transcription of genes such as annexin 1 (lipocortin 1), IL-10, IL-1 receptor antagonist, and IκBα, an inhibitor of nuclear factor-kappa B (NFκB). Glucocorticoids inhibit the transcription of both activating protein-1 (AP-1) and signal transducer activator of transcription 5 (STAT5). The most striking effect of the glucocorticoids is their ability to inhibit the expression of multiple inflammatory genes, including cytokines (IL-1, IL-2, IL-3, IL-4, IL-5, IL-6, IL-9, IL-11, IL-12, IL-13, and IL-16), chemokines (IL-8, MCP-1, -3, -4, and eotaxins), adhesion molecules (ICAM-1, VCAM-1, and E-selectin), enzymes (iNOS and Phos A2), and inflammatory receptors (NK1 receptors) [14].

2.3. Physiological Functions

GCs are essential for the maintenance of hemorrhagic states, infections and metabolic disturbances. GCs exert a variety of metabolic effects, such as the inhibition of glucose uptake, the stimulation of hepatic gluconeogenesis, and the increase of circulating glucose levels by peripheral tissues. Furthermore, GCs help in the maintenance of circulation, the induction of vascular tone and the increase of salt and water retention [21, 22, 23].

2.4. Therapeutic Use

The anti-inflammatory actions of therapeutic glucocorticoids are well known and are commonly used to treat diverse inflammatory conditions [22]. Various synthetic glucocorticoid molecules are available for therapeutic use [18].

Box 1. Therapeutic uses of glucocorticoids

Replacement therapy

- **Acute adrenal insufficiency**
- **Chronic adrenal insufficiency**
- **Congenital adrenal hyperplasia**

Non-endocrine diseases

- **Rheumatic disorders** (lupus erythematous, polyarteritis nodosa, Churg-Strauss syndrome, giant cell arteritis, rheumatoid arthritis)
- **Renal diseases** (nephrotic syndrome, glomerulonephritis, sclerosis)
- **Pulmonary diseases** (allergies, bronchial asthma, chronic obstructive pulmonary disease [COPD])
- **Infectious diseases** (*Haemophilus influenzae* type b meningitis)
- **Gastrointestinal diseases** (chronic ulcerative colitis, Crohn's disease)
- **Hepatic diseases** (autoimmune hepatitis)
- **Malignances** (chemotherapy, lymphocytic leukemia, lymphoma)
- **Other conditions** (sarcoidosis, thrombocytopenia, organ transplantation)

2.5. Glucocorticoids and Infections

Glucocorticoids are powerful drugs used to treat numerous diseases; however, the immunosuppression resulting from glucocorticoid use can lead to the reactivation of latent infectious diseases, such as tuberculosis [24], histoplasmosis [25], Chagas' disease [26], toxoplasmosis [27], leishmaniasis [28], cryptosporidiosis [29], amebiasis [30] and strongyloidiasis [31, 32].

GCs have a strong association with strongyloidiasis, particularly with the development of hyperinfection syndrome and dissemination. Hyperinfection syndrome has been observed regardless of the dose, duration, or route of administration of corticosteroids [33].

3. Strongyloides Stercoralis

3.1. Biology of *Strongyloides*

Fifty-two species of *Strongyloides* have been described in different hosts. In humans, the most common infectious species is *S. stercoralis.* Other species, such as *S. fuelleborni,* are found in Africa and Papua New Guinea. The worm has a complex life cycle in humans and animals. The obligate pulmonary phase of the life cycle typically occurs within hours of infection. Initiation of infection occurs when the infective third-stage larvae (L3) penetrate the skin and travel through the bloodstream to the lungs, where they migrate into the alveolar spaces, ascend the respiratory tree, and are swallowed. The larvae subsequently continue their development in the small intestine [3].

After passage through the lungs, the worms migrate to the intestine, where they develop into parthenogenetic females (a slender nematode from 1.5 to 10 mm in length); these females are capable of reproducing in the absence of males and lay embryonated eggs (60 μm in length). The first-stage larvae emerge from the hatching eggs, migrate into the intestinal lumen, and pass out of the host in the feces. In an external environment, the rhabditiform larvae (210 μm) differentiate into free-living female (small-bodied, up to 1.5 mm long by 85 μm wide) and male (slightly smaller than female worms, up to 1.2 mm) worms, or they may molt directly into third-stage larvae (600 μm in length) [34, 35].

3.2. Pathogenesis

The obligate pulmonary phase of the life cycle typically occurs within hours of infection, resulting in eosinophilic inflammation, mucus production, increased immunoglobulin production, and smooth muscle hyper-responsiveness [36, 37, 38]. After passing through the lungs, the worms migrate to the intestine, where they develop into females [39, 40] and induce intestinal eosinophilia and mastocytosis, both of which are thought to contribute to the process of worm elimination [41, 42].

The immune response is predominantly a Th2-type response characterized by high leukocyte recruitment and the overproduction of interleukin cytokines (IL-4, IL-5 and IL-13). Conversely, Th1-type responses are down-regulated during nematode infection [43, 44, 45, 46].

3.3. Hyperinfection Syndrome

The intestinal nematode *S. stercoralis* can persist in a human host for decades after the initial infection and can progress to a fulminant hyperinfection syndrome in immunocompromised hosts, particularly in patients who receive chronic corticosteroid treatment. Hyperinfection syndrome is an accelerated form of autoinfection resulting in an increased number of worms that disseminate into the extraintestinal regions: the mortality rate of hyperinfection syndrome is above 80% [3]. However, the pathophysiological basis of corticosteroid-enhanced risk for hyperinfection remains unclear.

Glucocorticoids are commonly prescribed drugs with effective immunosuppressive properties; however, their use is also a major risk factor for the progression of chronic strongyloidiasis to hyperinfection [47]. The incidence of hyperinfection syndrome has increased significantly with the use of glucocorticoids to treat several diseases that are considered immunological abnormalities, including lymphoma, lupus, rheumatoid arthritis, leprosy, asthma, COPD, polymyositis, and organ transplantation. Glucocorticoids are also used to treat intercurrent illnesses, such as Human T Lymphotropic Virus Type 1 (HTLV-1) and *Human Immunodeficiency Virus* (HIV) [8].

Glucocorticoids affect the immune response in a host by inhibiting the mast cell response and reducing circulating eosinophils, basophils, and monocytes. In addition, glucocorticoids enhance the apoptosis of eosinophils and lymphocytes [4, 11].

A new hypothesis was proposed in 1992 by Genta, suggesting that glucocorticoids have a direct effect on female worms. Ecdysis (molting in insects) is controlled by steroid molting hormones, known as ecdysteroids, which are produced in adult females. The glucocorticoids may occupy ecdysteroid receptors in the parasites (which exist in an unbound state under physiological conditions), and act as promoters of the molting process [13]. A report by Siddiqui et al describes a nuclear hormone receptor for a steroid/thyroid hormone in *S. stercoralis* larvae. The presence of such a receptor in *S. stercoralis* supports the hypothesis that steroids directly affect the parasite and may trigger the hyperinfection syndrome [48].

4. Experimental Model of Hyperinfection Syndrome Strongyloidiasis

To study the mechanisms underlying dexamethasone-induced alterations in the natural cycle of human strongyloidiasis (which is caused predominantly by *S. stercoralis*), we utilized a well-characterized rodent model of infection with *Strongyloides venezuelensis*. *S. venezuelensis* is a parasite that evokes a similar immune response to *S. stercoralis* in rodents [49] but is safer for use in the laboratory than *S. stercoralis*. We therefore infected rats with *S. venezuelensis* and treated them daily with dexamethasone.

4.1. Materials and Methods

SPF (Specific Pathogen-Free) male Wistar rats weighing 160 to 180 g, were used in the experiments. The rats were divided into three groups: uninfected animals, infected animals (Sv+PBS) and infected-treated animals (Sv+Dexa) were euthanized on 1, 3, 5, 7, 14 and 21 days post-infection (dpi). The second group was infected with $9x10^3$ larvae of *S. venezuelensis* and was administered daily with PBS (Phosphate buffered saline). The third group was infected and treated with 2 mg/kg daily of dexamethasone disodium phosphate (Dexa, Decadron®, Aché Laboratories, Campinas, Brazil). The infection procedure was previously described [50].

The collection of blood, bronchoalveolar lavage fluid (BALF) and peritoneal cavity fluid (PCF) was performed on days 1, 3, 5, 7, 14, and 21 post-infection. The chest cavity of each animal was opened, and the trachea was exposed and catheterized. The catheter was tied into place, and sterile PBS/sodium citrate was infused into the catheter. The PCF was obtained by injecting and withdrawing 5 ml of PBS into the peritoneal cavity. Total cell counts in blood, BALF and PCF were performed immediately upon harvest in a Neubauer chamber. Differential counts were obtained using Rosenfeld staining [51]. The lungs, spleen, kidney, heart, liver, and brain were harvested, minced and incubated so that migrating larvae could be collected and counted.

To histopathological analysis the lungs were inflated with 10% buffered formalin, immersed in this fixative for 48 h. Duodena were fixed in 10% buffered formalin. Sections were obtained, processed for paraffin embedding, and stained with hematoxilin and eosin (HE). Enzyme-linked immunosorbent assays (ELISA) were used to determine the levels of interleukin 1- beta (IL1-β) and IL-4. Tissue samples were homogenized and centrifuged and the supernatants were stored at -70°C until the assays were analyzed. The cytokine levels were determined according to the manufacturer's instructions (BD Pharmingen).

Sensitivities were >10 pg/mL. To extract infective larvae and female parasites for corticosterone analysis, cultures of rat feces and adult female parasites recovered from the small intestine of the Sv + Dexa group of rats were placed in sterile saline and centrifuged. Samples from untreated rats were obtained on day 7 post-infection, while dexamethasone-treated rats were harvested on days 7, 14 and 21 post-infection. The small parasite numbers recovered on days 14 and 21 in the Sv + PBS group did not allow for an appropriate comparison with the Sv + Dexa group. We therefore compared only the recovered larvae on days 7, 14 and 21 after dexamethasone treatment. After washing with saline and antibiotics 10 times, 5,000 adult female parasites and 20,000 larvae were incubated in 6-well plates with fungicide. The samples were then centrifuged for 5 min, the supernatants collected, and the parasites were homogenized with radioimmunoassay (RIA) buffer. The samples were centrifuged, and the supernatants were collected for the corticosterone assay.

Corticosterone levels were evaluated with an anti-corticosterone antibody (AB-Cort-17984) as previously reported in cultured supernatant and in RIA-homogenized samples after ethanol extraction from both infective larvae and female parasites [52]. For ecdysteroid quantification, infective larvae and adult female parasites were recovered from fecal cultures of infected rats treated with PBS or dexamethasone. Cultures were resuspended in saline and centrifuged. Samples from untreated rats were prepared on day 7 post-infection, while Sv + Dexa rats were harvested on days 7, 14 and 21 post-infection. The small parasite numbers recovered on days 14 and 21 in the Sv + PBS group prevented a direct comparison with the Sv + Dexa rats. Therefore, we compared only the recovered larvae on days 7, 14 and 21 after dexamethasone treatment. After parasite quantification, the supernatant was discarded and the pellet was weighed. For extraction of ecdysteroids, 1 ml of methanol was added to each sample. Supernatants were used for ecdysteroid quantification.

Antiserum produced in rabbits injected with a hemisuccinate derivative of ecdysone conjugated at C-22 was used for the ecdysteroid radioimmunoassay [53]. The methanol extracts were dried by centrifugation, and 100 μl of the radioactive ligand/antibody solution was added. The samples were incubated overnight at 4°C. The equilibrium reaction was terminated by adding 50% ammonium sulfate.

The precipitate was pelleted by centrifugation and then washed with ammonium sulfate. The pellet was subsequently dissolved in 40 μl of distilled water before adding 5 ml of HiSafe3 Optiphase LSC cocktail (Wallac-Packard) for liquid scintillation counting by a Beckman LS 6000 system. Assay conditions and cross reactivity factors for quantification of ecdysteroids and other compounds have previously been described [54, 55].

Because standard curves were established with the nonradioactive ligand 20-hydroxyecdysone (Simes, Milan), all results are expressed as 20E equivalents. Western immunoblot analysis was performed on homogenates obtained from larvae and adult female parasites, and the cytoplasmic fraction was obtained as reported by Kitchener [56]. Protein concentrations were determined by the Bradford method [57]. Rat hippocampus lysate was used as a positive control.

Proteins were denatured in Laemmli sample buffer for 5 min and then loaded onto a polyacrylamide gel. The proteins were transferred to PVDF membranes and blocked overnight with BSA.

Membranes were incubated for 2 hours with a polyclonal antibody to anti-glucocorticoid receptor. A peroxidase-conjugated anti-rabbit secondary antibody was applied. To detect immunoreactive bands, blots were incubated with a Pierce ECL chemiluminescence solution (Thermo Scientific, Rockford, Illinois, USA) followed by exposure to X-ray film as previously published [58].

4.2. Results

4.2.1. Dexamethasone Treatment of Infected Rats is Associated with Increased Parasite Burdens, Enhanced Female Worm Fertility, and Dissemination to Various Visceral Organs

Greater numbers of *S. venezuelensis* filariform larvae were recovered from Sv + Dexa-treated rat lungs starting at 1 dpi and reached a peak at 3 dpi. After 5 dpi, the numbers of larvae were reduced and no more larvae were recovered on day 21. Dexamethasone treatment initially exhibited a number of larvae similar to those of Sv + PBS-treated rats. However, the number of larvae in the Sv + Dexa rats was higher both 7 and 14 dpi when compared to the Sv + PBS group (Figure 1).

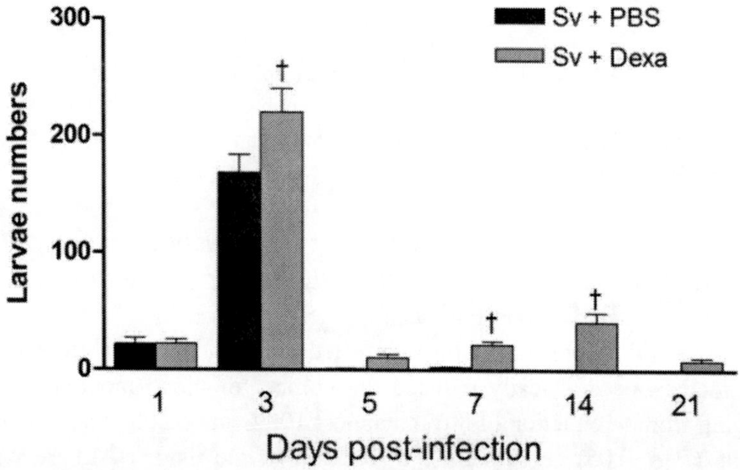

Figure 1. Number of larvae worms recovered from *Wistar* rats after *S. venezuelensis* infection. Rats were treated daily with PBS (Sv + PBS) or dexamethasone (Sv + Dexa). The lungs were tweezed in saline and maintained at 27°C for 2 h, followed by centrifugation, and the pellet was examined under light microscopy at a magnification of 50× to detect parasites. Data are expressed as the mean ± SEM (n = 5). $P < 0.05$; † Sv + PBS vs. Sv + Dexa.

Adult worms obtained from the intestines of Sv + PBS animals were analyzed through day 21; however, the parasites were almost completely eliminated from the intestine by that point in time. Conversely, the treatment with dexamethasone resulted in a significant increase in the number of adult female worms, particularly after day 7 and persisting through days 14 and 21 (Table 1).

The data in Table 2 suggest that daily treatment of infected rats with dexamethasone increased the number of infective larvae recovered from the spleen, kidney, heart, liver, and brain.

Table 1. Treatment with dexamethasone increases the number of adult worms observed in the duodena recovered after *S. venezuelensis* infection

	Number of adult worms	
Days	Sv + PBS	Sv + Dexa
5	3.2±0.5	4.5±0.5
7	3.6±0.3	4.7±0.4*
14	3.5±0.2	7.3±0.5*
21	0.6±0.3	6.0±0.7*

Duodenal sections were obtained 5, 7, 14, and 21 dpi. To evaluate the number of adult worms in histological slices, 10 fields were counted under light microscopy at a magnification of 100×. Data are expressed as the mean ± SEM. $P < 0.05$; * Sv + PBS vs. Sv + Dexa.

4.2.2. Dexamethasone Treatment Diminishes Eosinophil and Mononuclear Cell Counts in Blood, Lungs and Intestine.

The number of blood mononuclear cells in Sv + PBS rats were slightly increased when compared with uninfected animals; however, treatment with dexamethasone drastically reduced the number of blood mononuclear cells, ranging from a reduction of 80% to almost 100% among all experimental time points ($P < 0.05$) (Figure 2A). In relation to the lung, BALF revealed an increase in the number of mononuclear cells over the entire experimental period in Sv + PBS animals compared to uninfected animals. After dexamethasone treatment, the recruitment of mononuclear cells was significantly reduced. These levels were estimated at 50%, 46%, 45%, 25%, 30% and 5% at 1, 3, 5, 7, 14 and 21 days post-infection, respectively (Figure 2B). Finally, intestinal migration of the parasites was detected in Sv + PBS animals, with levels peaking on day 14. However, after dexamethasone treatment, the presence of the parasites was significantly diminished on days 1 (33%), 3 (35%), 5 (49%), 7 (52%), 14 (66%) and 21 (76%), $P < 0.05$ (Figure 2C). Sv + PBS rats developed systemic, pulmonary and peritoneal eosinophilia during all analyzed dates, consistent with a previous study in mice [38].

Table 2. Treatment with dexamethasone increases the number of infective larvae recovered from the lungs, spleen, kidney, heart, liver, and brain during *S. venezuelensis* infection

Days	Spleen		Kidney		Heart		Liver		Brain	
	Sv + PBS	Sv + Dexa	Sv + PBS	Sv + Dexa	Sv + PBS	Sv + Dexa	Sv + PBS	Sv + Dexa	Sv + PBS	Sv + Dexa
1	0	0	0	0	2±1.5	4±2	0	0	0±0	0
3	0.4±0.2	1±0.5	0.4±0.2	18±6*	2±0.7	5±2	0.6±0.4	1±0.4	0±0	0
5	0	0	0	0	0.8±0.6	1.2±0.6	0	0	0±0	0
7	0	0	0	2±0.7	0	1±0.3*	0.2±0.1	2±0.9	0±0	0
14	0	0	0	2±0.8	0	2±1	0.4±0.3	0.8±0.4	0±0	0.8±0.4
21	0	1±0.3	0	1±0.3	0	0.8±0.4	0	0.6±0.3	0±0	0.3±0.2

Spleen, kidney, heart, liver, and brain were obtained 1, 3, 5, 7, 14, and 21 dpi. To evaluate the number of infective larvae, the organs were minced in saline and maintained at 27°C for 2 h, followed by centrifugation, and the pellet was examined under light microscopy at a magnification of 50× to detect parasites. Data are expressed as the mean ± SEM. $P < 0.05$; * Sv + PBS vs. Sv + Dexa.

Sv + PBS animals also showed blood eosinophilia on the first day of infection, with a peak at day 7 and a progressive decrease in eosinophilia until day 21. Dexamethasone treatment completely inhibited blood eosinophilia at levels lower than uninfected animals throughout the entire experimental period ($P < 0.05$) (Figure 2D). In the Sv + PBS animals' BALF, eosinophil counts increased significantly from day 1 of the infection, with a peak at day 3, and decreased progressively to levels of eosinophils below the limit of detection on experimental days 14 and 21.

Although a similar behavior was observed upon dexamethasone treatment, eosinophil counts were extremely low in this case, showing reductions of 93%, 57%, 73% and 95% ($P < 0.05$) at days 1, 3, 5 and 7, respectively (Figure 2E). No eosinophils were detected in the BALF of uninfected animals. In the peritoneal cavity, the number of eosinophils was increased on the first day, peaked at day 14, and was reduced by day 21. Dexamethasone treatment drastically reduced eosinophil recruitment to the peritoneal cavity throughout the entire experiment ($P < 0.05$), exhibiting levels that were lower than those observed in uninfected rats (Figure 2F).

4.2.3. Histopathological Findings of S. venezuelensis *Infection and Dexamethasone Treatment*

In Sv + PBS animals, the major effects of parasitic infection were observed in the lungs and intestines, specifically the duodenum. By day 21 post-infection, these animals displayed a remarkably rapid resolution of the mechanical damage and inflammation caused by *S. venezuelensis* larvae migrating through the pulmonary parenchyma (Figure 3). In contrast, dexamethasone treatment during infection promoted more prominent and confluent hemorrhagic foci containing larvae and cuticles. After day 5, the inflammatory process was notably granulomatous in Sv + PBS animals, containing epithelioid cells, giant cells, and eosinophils, some of which entrapped larval fragments (Figure 3B). Hemosiderin-laden macrophages were observed to be dispersed throughout the alveolar parenchyma. In contrast, Sv + Dexa animals showed no granuloma formation at any time, although numerous hemosiderin-laden macrophages were observed and were dispersed throughout the alveolar parenchyma. By day 7 post-infection, the granulomas were defined and compact in Sv + PBS rats, whereas Sv + Dexa animals still did not show any evidence of granulomatous inflammation. After 14 days of infection, the granulomas were scarce and no parasites were visualized in Sv + PBS rats. Sv + Dexa animals continued to show dispersed macrophages, and free larvae were observed in the alveolar parenchyma (Figure 3I). Finally, on day 21, only residual granulomas and a minimal inflammatory infiltrate were observed in Sv + PBS and Sv + Dexa animals. These results were similar to those obtained on day 14; however, no more larvae were found. In uninfected animals, no apparent morphological alterations could be observed.

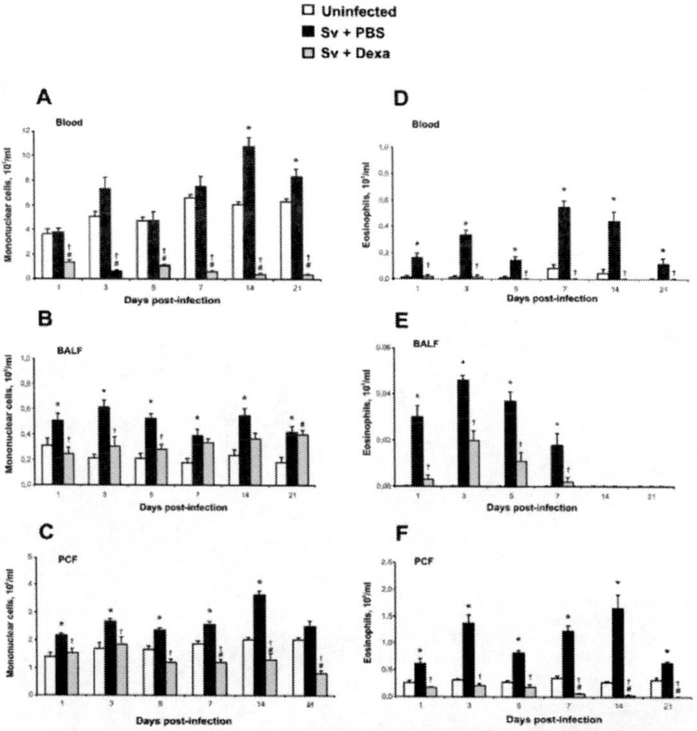

Figure 2. Levels of mononuclear cells (A, B and C) and eosinophils (D, E and F) in the blood, bronchoalveolar lavage fluid (BALF) and peritoneal cavity fluid (PCF). Cells were obtained after infection with *S. venezuelensis* (Sv) infective larvae. Rats were treated daily with vehicle (Sv + PBS) or dexamethasone (Sv + Dexa). A group of uninfected rats was used as a control. The numbers of mononuclear cells and eosinophils were identified through Rosenfeld staining. Data are expressed as the mean ± SEM (n = 5). $P < 0.05$; * Uninfected vs. Sv + PBS, #Uninfected vs. Sv + Dexa; †Sv + PBS vs. Sv + Dexa.

Beginning on day 3, adult parasites could be observed intermixed with abundant mucus in the intestinal lumen of both Sv + PBS and Sv + Dexa animals, accompanied by a submucosal mononuclear infiltrate containing few eosinophils. Females surrounded by slightly more prominent inflammatory infiltrates were observed on day 5 in both groups, although these infiltrates were more numerous in the Sv + Dexa animals (Figure 3Q). After 7 days, eosinophils were the most conspicuous cell present within the infiltrate, peaking by day 14 in Sv + PBS animals, whereas they were practically absent in Sv + Dexa animals. The most prominent inflammatory findings were on day 14. In addition to female worms, occasional epithelial erosions were observed in the Sv + PBS animals and were more numerous in the Sv + Dexa animals. Finally, the Sv + PBS animals showed a greater reduction in the number of female parasites and inflammatory infiltrates by day 21 post-infection, whereas in the Sv + Dexa animals, female parasites and damaged crypts were still observed. Uninfected animals showed no significant alterations in the intestinal mucosa. Histological examination of the other organs showed no evident morphological alterations (not shown).

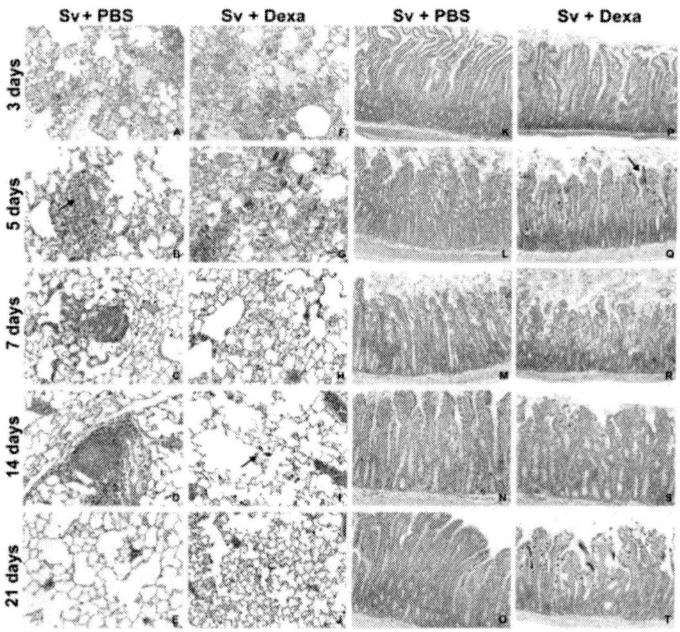

Figure 3. Histopathology of the lungs and duodena after infection with *S. venezuelensis* (Sv). Representative HE-stained 5-µm sections of lung and duodenal tissue of rats treated daily with vehicle (Sv + PBS) or dexamethasone (Sv + Dexa). Lungs of Sv + PBS rats are represented by panels A, B, C, D, and E. The arrow indicates the presence of a larva in the center of the granuloma (Figure 3B). The lungs of Sv + Dexa rats are shown in panels F, G, H, I, and J. The arrow indicates the presence of free larvae in the alveolar parenchyma (Figure 3I). The magnification of the panels is 200×. The duodena of Sv + PBS rats are represented by panels K, L, M, N, and O. The duodena of Sv + Dexa rats are shown in panels P, Q, R, S, and T. The arrow indicates the presence of an adult worm (Figure 3Q). The magnification of the panels is 100×.

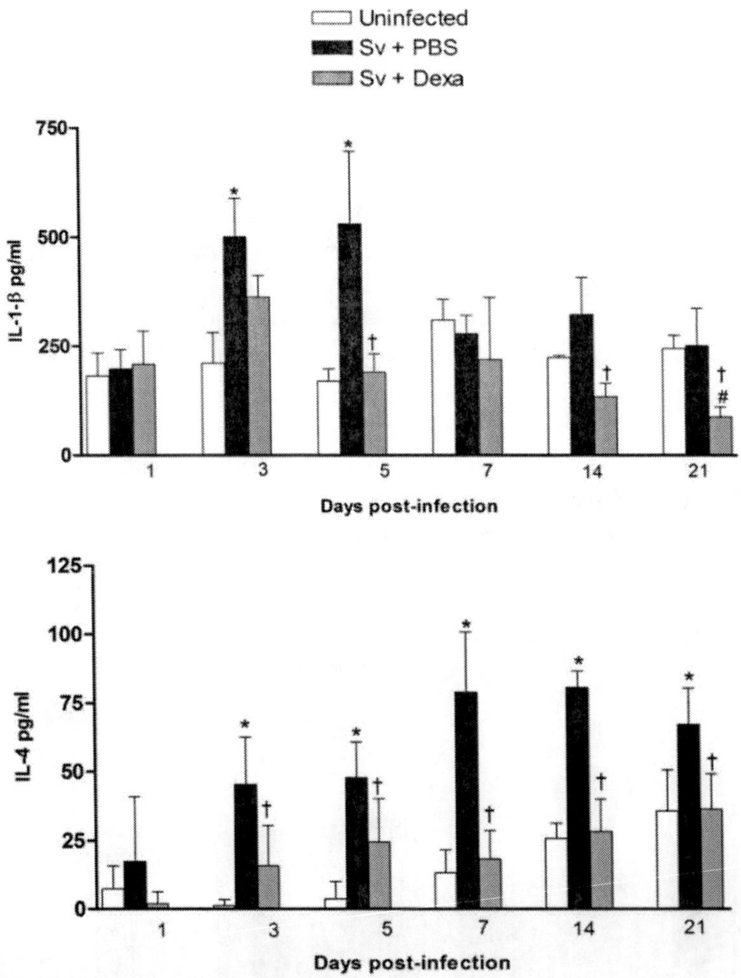

Figure 4. IL1-β and IL-4 in homogenized lung after infection with *S. venezuelensis.* Rats were treated daily with vehicle (Sv + PBS) or dexamethasone (Sv + Dexa). $P < 0.05$; *Uninfected vs. Sv + PBS, #Uninfected vs. Sv + Dexa; †Sv + PBS vs. Sv + Dexa.

4.2.4. Dexamethasone Treatment Diminishes Cytokine Levels during S. venezuelensis *Infection*

In Sv + PBS animals, the cytokine IL1-β showed a significant increase up until the 7th day after initial infection; however, the values subsequently diminished until day 21. The animals treated with dexamethasone displayed diminished levels of IL1-β overall in comparison with the Sv + PBS animals (*P*<0.05).

Furthermore, IL-4 production increased by day 3 and reached a peak on day 14. Dexamethasone treatment exhibited a significant reduction in IL-4 in comparison with the Sv + PBS group of rats (*P*<0.05); (Figure 4).

4.2.5. Dexamethasone Treatment Modulates the Production of Corticosterone by S. venezuelensis *Female Parasites and Infective Larvae*

Figures 5A and 5B show the corticosterone levels in the cultured supernatant of adult female parasites and infective larvae, respectively. There was no significant difference between the corticosterone levels in the infected rats exposed to dexamethasone or PBS 7 dpi. However, an increase in corticosterone production was observed in the cultured supernatant of adult female parasites recovered from dexamethasone-treated rats by 21 dpi when compared with the Sv + PBS group (Figure 5A). A similar trend was observed for the infective larvae supernatants recovered 21 dpi (Figure 5B).

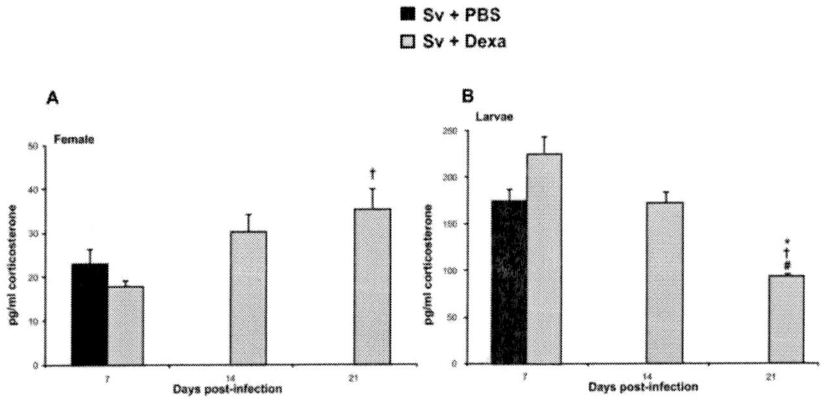

Figure 5. Levels of corticosterone in the supernatants of cultured female parasites (A) and infective larvae (B) obtained after infection with *S. venezuelensis* (Sv). Rats were treated daily with vehicle (Sv + PBS) or dexamethasone (Sv + Dexa). Corticosterone was measured by radioimmunoassay (RIA). Data are expressed as the mean ± SEM (n = 5). $P < 0.05$; *Comparison of 7 days (Sv + PBS) vs. 21 days (Sv + Dexa). †Comparison of 7 vs. 21 days in Sv + Dexa group. #Comparison of 14 vs. 21 days in the Sv + Dexa group.

4.2.6. Dexamethasone Treatment Leads to an Increase in Ecdysteroid Levels of S. venezuelensis *Adult Female Parasites and Infective Larvae*

Homogenates of adult female parasites (Figure 6A) and infective larvae (Figure 6B) were recovered from feces 7, 14, and 21 dpi and assayed for levels of an ecdysteroid-like material. At 7 dpi, the ecdysteroid levels measured in female parasite or larval extracts were similar in parasites recovered from PBS or dexamethasone-exposed rats. However, by 14 dpi, the ecdysteroid concentration had decreased in both female parasites and larvae recovered from PBS-treated rats and remained low until day 21. In contrast, adult and larval worms harvested from dexamethasone-treated rats showed detectable concentrations of ecdysteroids 14 and 21 post-infection. The ecdysteroid levels on day 21 were significantly higher than on days 7 or 14 (Figure 6A and 6B).

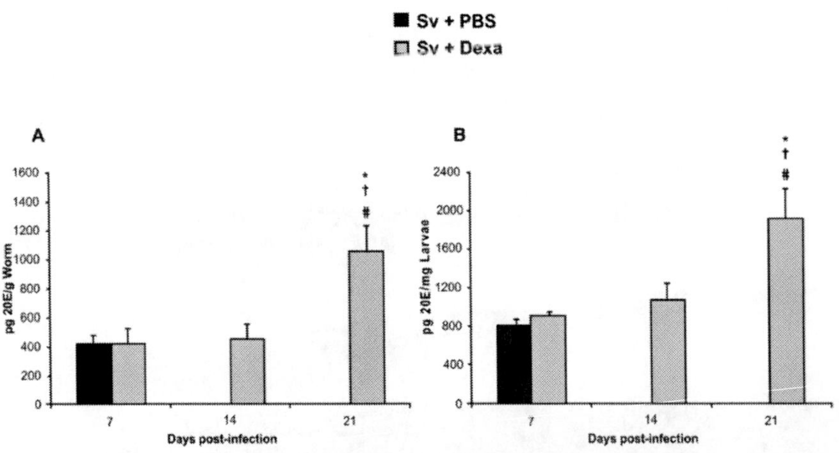

Figure 6. Levels of 20-hydroxyecdysone (ecdysterone or 20E) in homogenized female parasites (A) and infective larvae (B) obtained after infection with *S. venezuelensis* (Sv). Rats were treated daily with vehicle (Sv + PBS) or dexamethasone (Sv + Dexa). Ecdysterone was measured by radioimmunoassay (RIA). Data are expressed as the mean ± SEM (n = 5). $P < 0.05$; *Comparison of 7 days (Sv + PBS) vs. 21 days (Sv + Dexa). †Comparison of 7 vs. 21 days in Sv + Dexa group. #Comparison of 14 vs. 21 days in Sv + Dexa group.

4.2.7. Larvae and Adult Female Parasites Recovered from Infected Rats Express Glucocorticoid Receptor

Western blot analysis of a cytoplasmic extract from larvae revealed an approximately 94 kDa band representing glucocorticoid receptor expression. This band was not found in the female adult worm lysate. On the other hand, larvae and female worm extracts showed a strong band of a lower molecular weight (approximately 66 kDa) using the same polyclonal anti-glucocorticoid receptor antibody (Figure 7).

4.3. Discussion

In the present study, we have demonstrated that corticosteroid treatment induces a potent decrease in host immune response by reducing the number of eosinophils and mononuclear cells in multiple anatomical compartments. Importantly, dexamethasone treatment improved parasite fertility and proliferation and induced the dissemination of larvae to the lungs, spleen, kidneys, heart, liver, and brain, indicating hyperinfection. To the best of our knowledge, our data demonstrate for the first time that dexamethasone treatment leads to an increase in steroid hormone levels in *S. venezuelensis*, likely by increasing the synthesis of corticosterone and ecdysone-like hormones in adult females and larvae.

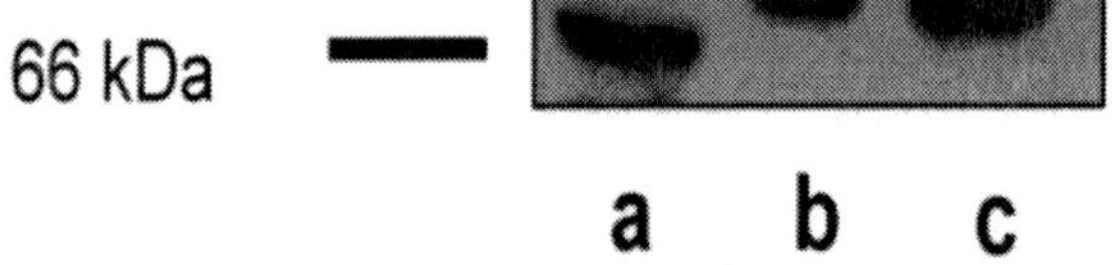

Figure 7. Analysis of glucocorticoid receptors. Proteins (20 μg) were obtained from *S. venezuelensis* adult female parasites and infective larvae. Cytoplasmic extracts were analyzed by Western immunoblot for the presence of glucocorticoid receptors. Lane (A) represents a positive control from a cytoplasmic fraction of a rat hippocampus lysate. Lane (B) represents a cytoplasmic extract from infective larvae, and lane (C) shows the cytoplasmic extract from an adult female.

The intestinal nematode *S. stercoralis* can persist in the human host for decades after initial infection and can progress into fulminant hyperinfection syndrome in immunocompromised hosts, particularly those receiving chronic corticosteroid treatment [8]. However, the pathophysiological mechanism of corticosteroid-enhanced risk for hyperinfection remains unclear. We used a rat model of strongyloidiasis to address this question. The pharmacological treatment of rats with dexamethasone interfered with several aspects of *S. venezuelensis* infection. Most notably, dexamethasone attenuated the inflammatory response in the major infected tissues (*i.e.*, lungs and intestines) and increased larval and adult persistence while enhancing female fertility. Infected animals that were not treated with steroids showed a remarkably rapid resolution of the mechanical damage and inflammation caused by larval migration through the pulmonary parenchyma. However, infected animals treated with dexamethasone showed prominent intra-alveolar hemorrhage containing numerous larvae and parasite cuticles.

These observations are similar to those observed in humans infected with *S. stercoralis.* Patients treated with corticosteroids exhibited an accelerated rate of autoinfection with dissemination of larvae to other organs [59, 60, 49]. Moreover, rhabditiform larvae could be recovered in the BALF of patients after chronic treatment with corticosteroids [61, 62]. Although these data do not offer a complete explanation, they do suggest that corticosteroids induce larvae to undergo more molts during their passage through the lungs, resulting in more parasite cuticles within the alveolar spaces [50]. Furthermore, corticosteroids may also directly induce the female worms to produce more eggs, which can result in an accelerated transformation of the rhabditiform larvae to the more invasive filariform larvae, thus promoting intense autoinfection and subsequent hyperinfection. Altogether, these effects appear to enhance nematode survival and to promote the dissemination of larvae to all tissues [4, 63, 64].

Dexamethasone treatment drastically reduced blood eosinophilia, which compromises eosinophil migration to the target-tissues. The current theory suggests that glucocorticoids most likely suppress eosinophil maturation by inhibiting the production and/or release of IL-5 and other eosinopoietic factors from cells within the bone marrow [65]. In addition to regulating the development of eosinophil infiltration, IL-5 may protect the host in a primary infection by limiting the number and fecundity of worms in the small intestine. IL-5 levels generally correlate with elevated blood and tissue eosinophilia in infected animals [66]. Moreover, glucocorticoids seem to reduce eosinophil accumulation at the site of inflammation by inhibiting the generation of chemoattractants and the upregulation of adhesion molecules [67, 68]. Interestingly, infected animals showed a different pattern in both mast cell and eosinophilic migration to the intestine; mast cells were conspicuous on day 3, whereas eosinophils peaked only at day 14. Dexamethasone also interfered in mast cell migration to the intestines, which likely compromises the functions related to the expulsion of the parasites [4, 69, 70]. Aside from inducing eosinophil recruitment, mast cells also inhibit attachment of the adult nematode to the intestinal epithelium, preventing subsequent invasion [71, 72, 73]. These inhibitory effects on eosinophil and mast cell tissue infiltration seem fundamental for the induction of hyperinfection [4, 74].

Strongyloides infection also promoted increased numbers of mononuclear cells in all compartments examined. Although conventionally associated with Th1-type responses, macrophage activation and the rapid recruitment of monocytes to infected tissue sites have been described during Th2-type responses to helminthes, providing an alternative source of IL-4, IL-13, IL-10 and IL-21 [75, 76]. In fact, the increases in IL-1 and IL-4 production were confirmed in our experiment. The mononuclear cells were highly elevated in the blood in our model, peaking on day 14 and decreasing slightly by day 21 of the experiment. Dexamethasone drastically inhibited mononuclear cell production, interfering with their migration to the lungs and intestines. In another study, using stereological analyses (a quantitative method that yields better spatial resolution of the inflammatory process), we demonstrated that most pulmonary macrophages are organized in granulomas around intrapulmonary larvae around the 5th day of infection [50]. Together with eosinophils, macrophages produce a delicate network of reticular fibers, mainly corresponding to collagen type III populations, which might be important in the host defense against intrapulmonary larvae [50, 77]. Dexamethasone treatment interfered significantly with this process, a claim supported by the fact that there were neither eosinophils nor well-developed granulomas in this group of rats. However, detached alveolar macrophages were found in the lung parenchyma, suggesting that eosinophils could play a pivotal role in granuloma organization [50, 77]. Nevertheless, further studies are necessary to elucidate the exact mechanism of granuloma formation in this parasitic infection. Another possible effect on the host immune system of dexamethasone treatment is the failure of antibody-dependent cellular cytotoxicity, which is one of the mechanisms responsible for parasite elimination [78, 79]. In this mechanism, eosinophils and mononuclear cells work as effector cells that attach to and release toxic molecules in the parasites after binding to specific antibodies covering the parasite surface [80, 81]. Because we did not measure antibody-dependent cellular cytotoxicity, this mechanism remains speculative.

By measuring ecdysteroid levels in extracts of larvae and female parasites, we attempted to address the question of physiological mechanisms underlying the observed hyperinfection. We showed that dexamethasone has a long lasting effect on the ecdysteroid levels of both larvae and adult female parasites. This finding indicates that dexamethasone may lead to hyperinfection by modulating ecdysteroid production in larvae and adult females, promoting the occurrence of molts in the larval stages and/or increased egg production in the female adults. Such a hypothesis, based on considerations by Genta [13] and Concha [4], is consistent with the identification of nuclear receptor genes in nematodes that are orthologs to insect nuclear receptors involved in the ecdysone response [48, 82, 83]. An interaction of corticosteroid nuclear receptors with the ecdysone signaling pathway induced by dexamethasone treatment could be a feasible mechanism to at least partially explain the observed hyperinfection.

In this study, we also demonstrated that nematode larvae expressed an immunoreactive band to the anti-glucocorticoid receptor antibody, whereas adult parasites did not, suggesting a direct action of dexamethasone on larval metabolism. It is interesting to note that the glucocorticoid receptor polyclonal antibody recognizes a strong band of a lower molecular weight (~66 kDa) both in larvae and adult female worms as well as in the positive control. This band could be a result of GR degradation or could represent crossreactivity with an as yet unidentified protein; however, this conclusion would require further study. Lethal human cases related to the development of hyperinfection after corticosteroid therapy in asymptomatic or mild strongyloidiasis have been reported [84, 85], pointing to the need of a better understanding of the mechanisms involved.

Conclusion

Our investigation was conducted to clarify the mechanism by which dexamethasone induces hyperinfection and dissemination of *Strongyloides* in an experimental model utilizing a natural host of this nematode. We observed that in addition to decreasing leukocyte numbers and possibly antibody-dependent cytotoxicity, dexamethasone treatment also increased larval ecdysone and female fertility. To the best of our knowledge, this is the first report demonstrating this phenomenon in response to corticosteroid therapy.

Ongoing studies are being conducted to more fully understand the effects of dexamethasone on *S. venezuelensis* infection.

Acknowledgments

The authors thank Elaine Medeiros Floriano and Carlos A. Sorgi for technical assistance. This work was supported by grants from the Fundação de Amparo à Pesquisa do Estado de São Paulo (FAPESP) (03/05469-5). SGR, LHF and MC are a research scientist at CNPq.

References

[1] Siddiqui, AA; Berk, SL. Diagnosis of *Strongyloides stercoralis* infection. *Clin Infect Dis*, 2001 33, 1040-47.

[2] Matsuda, K; Kim, BS; Whang, IS; Lim, CW; Baek, BK. Migration of *Strongyloides venezuelensis* in rats after oral inoculation of free-living infective larvae. *J Vet Med Sci*, 2003 65, 971-75.

[3] Grove, DI. Strongyloidiasis: a conundrum for gastroenterologists. *Gut*, 1994 35, 437-40.

[4] Concha, R; Harrington, WJr; Rogers, AI. Intestinal strongyloidiasis: recognition, management, and determinants of outcome. *J Clin Gastroenterol*, 2005 39, 203-11.

[5] Olsen, A; van Lieshout, L; Marti, H; Polderman, T; Polman, K; Steinmann, P; Stothard, R; Thybo, S; Verweij, JJ; Magnussen, P. Strongyloidiasis - the most neglected of the neglected tropical diseases? *Trans R Soc Trop Med Hyg*, 2009 103, 967-72.

[6] Viney, ME; Lok, JB. *Strongyloides* spp. WormBook, 2007 23, 1-15.

[7] Mokaddas, EM; Shati, S; Abdulla, A; Nampoori, NR; Iqbal, J; Nair, PM; Said, T; Abdulhalim, M; Hira, PR. Fatal strongyloidiasis in three kidney recipients in Kuwait. *Med Princ Pract*, 2009 18, 414-17.

[8] Keiser, PB; Nutman, TB. *Strongyloides stercoralis* in the immunocompromised population. *Clin Microbiol Rev*, 2004 17, 208-17.

[9] Schaeffer, MW; Buell, JF; Gupta, M; Conway, GD; Akhter, SA; Wagoner, LE. *Strongyloides* hyperinfection syndrome after heart transplantation: case report and review of the literature. *J Heart Lung Transplant,* 23 2004, 905-11.

[10] Pacanowski, J; Santos, M; Roux, A; Maignan, CL; Guillot, J; Lavarde, V; Cornet, M. Subcutaneous ivermectin as a safe salvage therapy in *Strongyloides stercoralis* hyperinfection syndrome: A case report. *Am J Trop Med Hyg*, 2005 73, 122-24.

[11] Genta, RM. Global prevalence of strongyloidiasis: critical review with epidemiologic insights into the prevention of disseminated disease. *Rev Infect Dis*, 1989 11, 755-67.

[12] Husni, RN; Gordon, SM; Longworth, DL; Adal, KA. Disseminated *Strongyloides stercoralis* infection in an immunocompetent patient. *Clin Infect Dis*, 1996 23, 663.

[13] Genta, RM. Dysregulation of strongyloidiasis: a new hypothesis. *Clin Microbiol Rev*, 1992 5, 345-55.

[14] Barnes, PJ. Molecular mechanisms and cellular effects of glucocorticosteroids. *Immunol Allergy Clin North Am*, 2005 25, 451-68.

[15] Schimmer, BP; Parker, KL. Adrenocorticotropic hormone; adrenocortical steroids and their synthetic analogs; inhibitors of the synthesis and actions of adrenocortical hormones. In: Brunton, L; Lazo, J; Parker, K. Goodman & Gilman's. The Pharmacological Basis of Therapeutics. New York: McGraw-Hill; 2006; 11th ed.; p.1597.

[16] Fawcett, DW. Bloom and Fawcett a Textbook of Histology. New York: Chapman and Hall; 1994; 12th ed.; p. 988.

[17] Barnes, PJ. Mechanisms and resistance in glucocorticoid control of inflammation. *J Steroid Biochem Mol Biol*, 2010 120, 76-85.

[18] McMaster, A; Ray, DW. Modelling the glucocorticoid receptor and producing therapeutic agents with anti-inflammatory effects but reduced side-effects. *Exp Physiol*, 2007 92, 299-309.

[19] Pu, Z; Krugers, HJ; Joëls, M. Corticosterone time-dependently modulates beta-adrenergic effects on long-term potentiation in the hippocampal dentate gyrus. *Learn Mem*, 2007 14, 359-67.

[20] Adcock, IM; Barnes, PJ. Molecular mechanisms of corticosteroid resistance. *Chest*, 2008 134, 394-401.

[21] Munck, A; Holbrook, NJ. Glucocorticoid-receptor complexes in rat thymus cells. Rapid kinetic behavior and a cyclic model. *J Biol Chem*, 1984 259, 820-31.

[22] Wilckens, T. Glucocorticoids and immune function: physiological relevance and pathogenic potential of hormonal dysfunction. *Trends Pharmacol Sci*, 1995 16, 193-97.

[23] Hardy, RS; Raza, K; Cooper, MS. Endogenous glucocorticoids in inflammation: contributions of systemic and local responses. *Swiss Med Wkly*, 2012 142, w13650.

[24] Jick, SS; Lieberman, ES; Rahman, MU; Choi, HK. Glucocorticoid use, other associated factors, and the risk of tuberculosis. *Arthritis Rheum*, 2006 55, 19-26.

[25] Arunkumar, P; Crook, T; Ballard, J. Disseminated histoplasmosis presenting as pancytopenia in a methotrexate-treated patient. *Am J Hematol*, 2004 77, 86-87.

[26] Rassi, A; Amato Neto, V; de Siqueira, AF; Doles, J; Leite, MS; Silva, OQ; Cardoso, VM. The influence of corticoids, in Chronic Chagas disease, administered in virtue of associated disorders. *Rev Soc Bras Med Trop*, 1997 30, 93-99.

[27] Chinchilla, M; Guerrero, OM; Reyes, L; Castro, A. Effect of corticosteroids on the congenital transmission of experimental toxoplasmosis. *Rev Biol Trop*, 1992 40, 135-37.

[28] Gangneux, JP; Chau, F; Sulahian, A; Derouin, F; Garin, YJ. Effects of immunosuppressive therapy on murine *Leishmania infantum* visceral leishmaniosis. *Eur Cytokine Netw*, 1999 10, 557-9.

[29] Adjei, AA; Jones, JT; Enriquez, FJ; Yamamoto, S. Dietary nucleosides and nucleotides reduce *Cryptosporidium parvum* infection in dexamethasone immunosuppressed adult mice. *Exp Parasitol*, 1999 92, 199-208.

[30] Abaza, SM; Makhlouf, LM; el-Shewy, KA; el-Moamly, AA. Intestinal opportunistic parasites among different groups of immunocompromised hosts. *J Egypt Soc Parasitol*, 1995 25, 713-27.

[31] Rodrigues, MA; Fróes, RC; Anefalos, A; Kobayasi, S. Invasive enteritis by *Strongyloides stercoralis* presenting as acute abdominal distress under corticosteroid therapy. *Rev Hosp Clin Fac Med Sao Paulo*, 2001 56, 103-06.

[32] Pagliuca, A. *Strongyloides* hyperinfection in adult T-cell leukaemia/lymphoma. *Br J Haematol*, 1999 105, 1.

[33] Mejia, R; Nutman, TB. Screening, prevention, and treatment for hyperinfection syndrome and disseminated infections caused by *Strongyloides stercoralis*. *Curr Opin Infect Dis*, 2012 25, 458-63.

[34] Schad, GA. Morphology and life history of *Strongyloides stercoralis*. In: Grove, DI. Strongyloidiasis a major roundworm infection of man. London, United Kingdom: Taylor and Francis; 1989; p. 85-104.

[35] Speare, R. Identification of species of *Strongyloides*. In: Grove, DI. Strongyloidiasis a major roundworm infection of man. London, United Kingdom: Taylor and Francis; 1989; p. 11-84.
[36] Allen, JE; Maizels, RM. Immunology of human helminth infection. *Int Arch Allergy Immunol*, 1996 109, 3-10.
[37] El-Malky, M; Maruyama, H; Hirabayashi, Y; Shimada, S; Yoshida, A; Amano, T; Tominaga, A; Takatsu, K; Ohta, N. Intraepithelial infiltration of eosinophils and their contribution to the elimination of adult intestinal nematode, *Strongyloides venezuelensis* in mice. *Parasitol Int*, 2003 52, 71-79.
[38] Machado, ER; Ueta, MT; Lourenço, EV; Anibal, FF; Sorgi, CA; Soares, EG; Roque-Barreira, MC; Medeiros, AI; Faccioli, LH. Leukotrienes play a role in the control of parasite burden in murine strongyloidiasis. *J Immunol*, 2005 175, 3892-99.
[39] Grove, DI. Human strongyloidiasis. *Adv Parasitol*, 1996 38, 251-309.
[40] Reece, JJ; Siracusa, MC; Scott, AL. Innate immune responses to lung-stage helminth infection induce alternatively activated alveolar macrophages. *Infect Immun*, 2006 74, 4970-81.
[41] Korenaga, M; Hitoshi, Y; Yamaguchi, N; Sato, Y; Takatsu, Y; Tada, I. The role of interleukin-5 in protective immunity to *Strongyloides venezuelensis* infection in mice. *Immunology*, 1991 72, 502-07.
[42] Machado, ER; Carlos, D; Lourenço, EV; Sorgi, CA; Silva, EV; Ramos, SG; Ueta, MT; Aronoff, DM; Faccioli, LH. Counterregulation of Th2 immunity by interleukin 12 reduces host defenses against *Strongyloides venezuelensis* infection. *Microbes Infect*, 2009 11, 571-78.
[43] Maizels, RM; Yazdanbakhsh, M. Immune regulation by helminth parasites: cellular and molecular mechanisms. *Nat Rev Immunol*, 2003 3, 733-44.
[44] Anthony, RM; Rutitzky, LI; Urban, JFJr; Stadecker, MJ; Gause, WC. Protective immune mechanisms in helminth infection. *Nat Rev Immunol*, 2007 7, 975-87.
[45] Machado, ER; Carlos, D; Lourenço, EV; Souza, GE; Sorgi, CA; Silva, EV; Ueta, MT; Ramos, SG; Aronoff, DM; Faccioli, LH. Cyclooxygenase-derived mediators regulate the immunological control of *Strongyloides venezuelensis* infection. *FEMS Immunol Med Microbiol,* 2010 59, 18-32.
[46] Iriemenam, NC; Sanyaolu, AO; Oyibo, WA; Fagbenro-Beyioku, AF. *Strongyloides stercoralis* and the immune response. *Parasitology International,* 2010 59, 9-14.

[47] Al Maslamani, MA; Al Soub, HA; Al Khal, AL; Al Bozom, IA; Abu Khattab, MJ; Chacko, KC. *Strongyloides stercoralis* hyperinfection after corticosteroid therapy: a report of two cases. *Annals of Saudi of Medicine*, 2009 29, 397-401.

[48] Siddiqui, AA; Stanley, CS; Skelly, PJ; Berk, SL. A cDNA encoding a nuclear hormone receptor of the steroid/thyroid hormone-receptor superfamily from the human parasitic nematode *Strongyloides stercoralis*. *Parasitol Res*, 2000 86, 24-29.

[49] Fardet, L; Généreau, T; Poirot, JL; Guidet, B; Kettaneh, A; Cabane, J. Severe strongyloidiasis in corticosteroid-treated patients: case series and literature review. *J Infect*, 2007 54, 18-27.

[50] Tefé-Silva, C; Souza, DI; Ueta, MT; Floriano, EM; Faccioli, LH; Ramos, SG. Interference of dexamethasone in the pulmonary cycle of *Strongyloides venezuelensis* in rats. *Am J Trop Med Hyg*, 2008 79, 571-78.

[51] Faccioli, LH; Souza, GE; Cunha, FQ; Poole, S; Ferreira, SH. Recombinant interleukin-1 and tumor necrosis factor induce neutrophil migration "in vivo" by indirect mechanisms. *Agents Actions*, 1990 30, 344-49.

[52] Laguna-Abreu, MTC; Margatho, L; Germano, CMR; Antunes-Rodrigues, J; Elias, LLK; Castro, M. The effect of adrenalectomy on Fos expression in vasopressinergic and oxytocinergic neurons in response to stress in the rat. *Stress*, 2007 10, 332-41.

[53] Warren, JT; Gilbert, LI. Ecdysone metabolism and distribution during the pupal adult development of *Manduca sexta*. *Insect Biochem*, 1986 16, 65-82.

[54] Feldlaufer, MF; Hartfelder, K. Relationship of the neutral sterols and ecdysteroids of the parasitic mite, *Varroa jacobsoni* to those of the honey bee, *Apis mellifera*. *J Insect Physiol*, 1997 43; 541-45.

[55] Basso, Jr LR; Vasconcelos, C; Fontes, AM; Hartfelder, K; Silva, JrJA; Coelho, PSR; Monesi, N; Paçó-Larson, ML. The induction of DNA puff *BhC4-1* gene is a late response to the increase in 20-hydroxyecdysone titers in last instar dipteran larvae. *Mech Dev*, 2002 110, 15-26.

[56] Kitchener, P; Blassi, FD; Borreli, E; Piazza, PV. Differences between brain structures in nuclear translocation and DNA binding of the glucocorticoid receptor during stress and the circadian cycle. *Eur J Neurosc*, 2004 19, 1837-46.

[57] Bradford, MM. A rapid and sensitive method for the quantitation of microgram quantities of protein utilizing the principle of protein-dye binding. *Anal Biochem*, 1976 7, 248-54.

[58] Castro, M; Elliot, S; Kino, T; Bamberger, C; Karl, M; Webster, E; Chrousos, GP. The non-ligand binding ß-isoform of human glucocorticoid receptor (hGRß): tissue levels, mechanism of action and potential physiologic role. *Mol Med*, 1996 2, 597-607.

[59] Smith, B; Verghese, A; Guiterrez, C; Dralle, W; Berk, SL. Pulmonary strongyloidiasis. Diagnosis by sputum gram stain. *Am J Med,* 1985 79, 663-66.

[60] Yee, A; Boylen, CT; Noguchi, T; Klatt, EC; Sharma, OP. Fatal *Strongyloides stercoralis* infection in a patient receiving corticosteroids. *West J Med*, 1987 146, 363-64.

[61] Williams, J; Nunley, D; Dralle, W; Berk, SL; Verghese, A. Diagnosis of pulmonary strongyloidiasis by bronchoalveolar lavage. *Chest*, 1988 94, 643-44.

[62] Aregawi, D; Lopez, D; Wick, M; Scheld, WM; Schiff, D. Disseminated strongyloidiasis complicating glioblastoma therapy: a case report. *J Neurooncol*, 2009 94, 439-43.

[63] Neva, FA. Biology and immunology of human strongyloidiasis. *J Infect Dis*, 1986 153, 397-406.

[64] Guyomard, JL; Chevrier, S; Bertholom, JL; Guigen, C; Charlin, JF. Finding of *Strongyloides stercoralis* infection, 25 years after leaving the endemic area, upon corticotherapy for ocular trauma. *J Fr Ophtalmol*, 2007 30, e4.

[65] Barnes, PJ. Anti-inflammatory mechanisms of glucocorticoids. *Biochem Soc Trans*, 1995 23, 940-45.

[66] Ovington, KS; McKie, K; Matthaei, KI; Young, IG; Behm, CA. Regulation of primary *Strongyloides ratti* infections in mice: a role for interleukin-5. *Immunology*, 1998 95, 488-93.

[67] Belvisi, MG. Regulation of inflammatory cell function by corticosteroids. *Proc Am Thorac Soc,* 2004 1, 207-14.

[68] ten Hove, W; Houben, LA; Raaijmakers, JA; Koenderman, L; Bracke, M. Rapid selective priming of FcalphaR on eosinophils by corticosteroids. *J Immunol*, 2006 177, 6108-14.

[69] Trajman, A; MacDonald, TT; Elia, CC. Intestinal immune cells in S*trongyloides stercoralis* infection. *J Clin Pathol*, 1997 50, 991-95.

[70] Wilkes, CP; Bleay, C; Paterson, S; Viney, ME. The immune response during a *Strongyloides ratti* infection of rats. *Parasite Immunol*, 2007 29, 339-46.

[71] Miller, HR; Huntley, JF; Wallace, GR. Immune exclusion and mucus trapping during the rapid expulsion of *Nippostrongylus brasiliensis* from primed rats. *Immunology*, 1981 44, 419-29.

[72] Brigandi, RA; Rotman, HL; Leon, O; Nolan, TJ; Schad, GA; Abraham, D. *Strongyloides stercoralis* host-adapted third-stage larvae are the target of eosinophil-associated immune-mediated killing in mice. *J Parasitol*, 1998 84, 440-45.

[73] Maruyama, H; Yabu, Y; Yoshida, A; Nawa, Y; Ohta, N. A role of mast cell glycosaminoglycans for the immunological expulsion of intestinal nematode, *Strongyloides venezuelensis*. *J Immunol*, 2000 164, 3749-54.

[74] Mansfield, LS; Niamatali, S; Bhopale, V; Volk, S; Smith, G; Lok, JB; Genta, RM; Schad, GA. *Strongyloides stercoralis*: maintenance of exceedingly chronic infections. *Am J Trop Med Hyg*, 1996 55, 617-24.

[75] Gordon, S. Alternative activation of macrophages. Nat Rev Immunol, 2003 3, 23-35.

[76] Siracusa, MC; Reece, JJ; Urban, JFJr; Scott, AL. Dynamics of lung macrophage activation in response to helminth infection. *J Leukoc Biol*, 2008 84, 1422-33.

[77] Lenzi, HL; Kimmel, E; Schechtman, H; Pelajo-Machado, M; Vale, BS; Panasco, MS; Lenzi, JÁ. Collagen arrangement in hepatic granuloma in mice infected with *Schistosoma mansoni*: dependence on fiber radiation centers. *Braz J Med Biol Res*, 1999 32, 639-43.

[78] Ligas, JÁ; Kerepesi, LA; Galioto, AM; Lustigman, S; Nolan, TJ; Schad, GA; Abraham, D. Specificity and mechanism of immunoglobulin M (IgM)- and IgG-dependent protective immunity to larval *Strongyloides stercoralis* in mice. *Infect Immun*, 2003 71, 6835-43.

[79] Machado, ER; Ueta, MT; Lourenço, EV; Anibal, FF; Roque-Barreira, MC; Faccioli, LH. Comparison of immune responses in mice infected with different strains of *Strongyloides venezuelensis*. *Parasite Immunol*, 2007 29, 549-57.

[80] Dombrowicz, D; Capron, M. Eosinophils, allergy and parasites. *Curr Opin Immunol*, 2001 13, 716-20.

[81] Pearce, EJ; MacDonald, AS. The immunobiology by schistosomiasis. *Nat Rev Immunol*, 2002 2, 499-511.

[82] Crossgrove, K; Laudet, V; Maina, CV. *Dirofilaria immitis* encoded Di-nhr-7, a putative orthologue of the *Drosophila* ecdysone-regulated E78 gene. *Mol Biochem Parasitol*, 2002 119, 169-77.

[83] Shea, C; Hough, D; Xiao, JP; Tzertzinis, G; Maina, GV. An rxr/usp homolog from the parasitic nematode *Dirofilaria immitis*. *Gene*, 2004 324, 171-18.

[84] Orlent, H; Crawley, C; Cwynarski, K; Dina, R; Apperley, J. Strongyloidiasis pre and post autologous peripheral blood stem cell transplantation. *Bone Marrow Transplant*, 2003 32, 115-17.

[85] Reddy, IS; Swarnalata, G. Fatal disseminated strongyloidiasis in patients on immunosuppressive therapy: report of two cases. *Indian J Dermatol Venereol Leprol*, 2005 71, 38-40.

In: Dexamethasone
Editors: A. Sauvage and M. Levy
ISBN: 978-1-62808-405-4

Chapter III

Dexamethasone's Uses in Retinal Diseases

***Zeljka Smit-McBride*[1,*]*, Sara P. Modjtahedi*[2] *and Lawrence S. Morse*[1]**
[1]University of California at Davis, School of Medicine, Department of Ophthalmology, Davis, CA, US
[2]Kaiser Permanente Medical Group, Sacramento, CA, US

Abstract

Steroids, having both anti-inflammatory and anti-angiogenic properties, are a useful therapeutic option in the treatment of retinal disease. Intravitreal steroids can be used in the treatment of various retinal conditions including diabetic and vasculo-occlusive macular edema, exudative macular degeneration, pseudophakic cystoid macular edema, and posterior uveitis. Although there are well known serious potential complications with intravitreal steroids, including glaucoma and endophthalmitis, recent studies have shown that intravitreal steroids may be used as a safe alternative to the practice of laser therapy for the treatment of macular edema secondary to diabetes or vein occlusions. Although there are several steroid formulations that may be used, this article focuses on the use of intravitreal dexamethasone. Dexamethasone

* E-mail: zsmcbride@ucdavis.edu.

is a potent anti-inflammatory agent that inhibits multiple inflammatory cytokines. Despite its established therapeutic benefit, side effects such as cataract formation and ocular hypertension/glaucoma raise concerns. Therefore, understanding the molecular and genetic effects of intraocular steroid treatments is of utmost importance and of clinical relevance. Our *in vivo* studies have elucidated several genes and pathways that are potentially altering the neuroprotective and/or neurodegenerative balance between glial and retinal ganglion cells during intravitreal steroid treatment, such as semaphorin signaling, a member of the neuronal axonal guidance signaling system. Furthermore, our more recent data results suggests that dexamethasone affects the balance of Th1, Th2 and Th17 cytokine production, which influences many pathological processes and plays both causative and protective roles in retinal disease.

Introduction

Steroids have both anti-inflammatory and anti-angiogenic properties, and thus are a mainstay therapeutic option in the ophthalmic practice. Intravitreal steroids can be used in the treatment of various potentially blinding retinal conditions including diabetic retinopathy, macular degeneration, vein occlusion, and non-infectious uveitis [1]. Despite the benefits of intravitreal steroids, there are several serious potential ocular complications—namely cataracts and glaucoma, that may require surgical intervention or even result in permanent vision loss. These complications limit the use of intravitreal steroids in certain patient populations. Although there are well known serious potential complications with intravitreal steroids, studies have shown that intravitreal steroids may be used as a safe alternative to the standard practice of laser therapy for the treatment of macular edema secondary to diabetes or vein occlusions [2]. Although there are several steroid formulations that may be used, this article focuses on the use of intravitreal dexamethasone, both in solution and implant-form.

Mechanism of Action

Endogenous Glucocorticoid Signaling

The main role in regulating signaling by glucocorticoid receptor (GR) is played by the hypothalamic-pituitary-adrenal axis. Neural, endocrine and cytokine signals are controlled via this axis which secretes the glucocorticoid, cortisol, in humans and corticosterone, in mice [3] and refs therein). The glucocorticoid receptor is a member of the nuclear steroid receptor superfamily (with mineralocorticoid, thyroid hormone, retinoic acid and vitamin D receptors) [4], and has a high affinity for cortisol. The GR is ubiquitously expressed in tissues, and regulates tissue specific gene expression of a multitude of target genes. These genes are involved in a diverse array of physiologic functions, such as tissue development, homeostatic regulation, suppression of inflammation and stress response induced by noise, restraint, hypoglycemic or immune challenge [5] and references therein). Figure 1 illustrates some of those pathways.

The GR can be functionally divided in several domains: a N-terminal transcription activation domain, a central DNA binding domain with Zn-fingers and a C-terminal ligand/steroid hormone binding domain. The glucocorticoid receptor is coded by only one gene with nine exons, evolutionarily highly conserved [6], but it has a multitude of variants present in the cells. First there are splice variants, which generate variants at the mRNA level. The main proteins translated from them are GRalpha, and a C-terminal variant GRbeta, which has a deletion of ligand/steroid hormone binding domain, that likely has a dominant negative effect on GRalpha. Less abundant and with less understood function are GRdelta, mainly expressed in cancer and GRgamma, with additional Arg in the DNA binding domain [7, 8]. Furthermore, there are multiple proteins translated from GRalpha transcripts, that use alternative translation initiation sites, and the GR is subject to a variety of posttranslational modifications, which adds to even larger diversity of GR proteins [8]. The GR protein variants have been shown to have differential activity on gene regulation, and have also been shown to have cell type specific differential expression.

Glucocorticoid hormone (GH) gets inside of cells by diffusion. GH diffuses across plasma membrane, binds to glucocorticoid receptors in the cytoplasm, and promotes its dissociation from chaperone proteins i.e., heat-shock proteins. Activated GRs can dimerize and translocate to the nucleus, where they bind to glucocorticoid response elements (GREs) in the promoter of glucocorticoid responsive genes, resulting in change in their transcription. This results in the increase of the transcription of genes that act to suppress inflammation, i.e. interleukin-1 receptor antagonist. Additional level of tissue specific regulation occurs from interaction of GR-GH complex with other, tissue specific transcription factors, such as proinflammatory NF-kappa B [9, 10], ICAM, or TNF∂ and MAPK pathways [11-14].

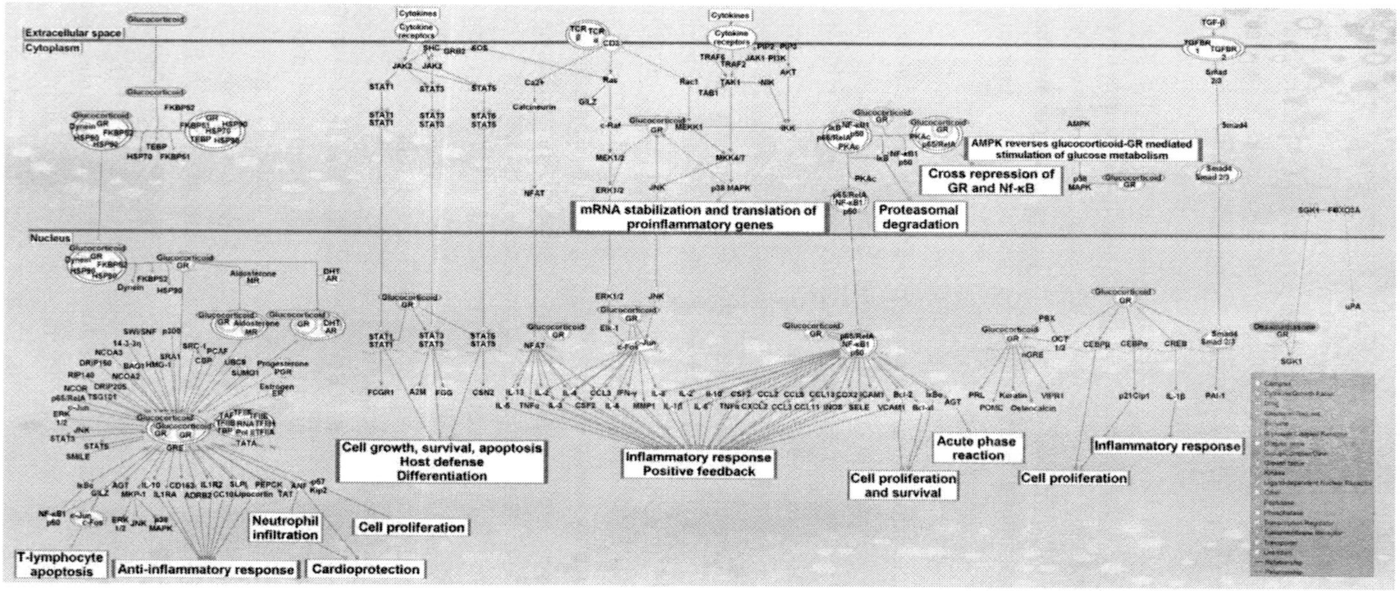

Figure 1. Glucocorticoids and glucocorticoid receptors are involved in regulation of a diverse array of biological pathways and physiologic functions.

These two mechanisms 1) direct transcriptional activation by binding to GRE and 2) interaction with other transcription factors, are often referred as classical GR mechanisms of action. Third, so called "rapid action" mechanism acts via so called non-genomic pathways, through membrane-associated receptors, such as G protein coupled receptors (GPRCs) and second messengers which activate several signal transduction pathways [15, 16]. And, yet, there are additional epigenetics modes of action that include histone deacetylation, leading to suppression of gene expression [11-13] and methylation. Systemic use of steroids has been shown to result in genome-wide alterations in promoter methylation [17, 18]. Some of these multiple modes of action of GR are depicted in Figure 2.

Synthetic Glucocorticoids

The synthetic glucocorticoids are the most potent anti-inflammatory agents known, but their use is limited owing to the range and severity of their side-effects. Although their structure is based on natural GR ligands, their chemical structure has been changed slightly to optimize therapeutic potential and minimize adverse reactions [19]. The studies of the structure of the ligand binding domain of the GR have shown that even subtle changes to the ligand structure alter the final conformation of the ligand–receptor complex, with dramatic consequences for the whole protein conformation, and function of the receptor [20-22].

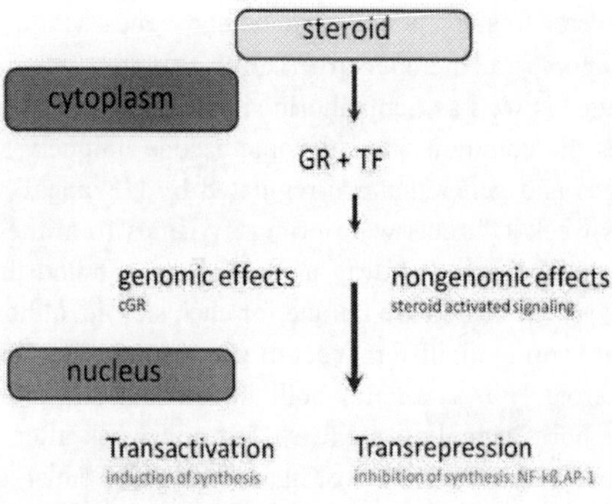

Figure 2. Multiple modes of action of glucocorticoids in the cell.

Expression Analysis of Dexamethasone in Ocular Tissue

While dexamethasone has a very efficient anti-inflammatory clinical effect, complications such as cataract formation and steroid induced glaucoma are common. The results of our study showed that while glucocorticoids stimulated many of anti-inflammatory and neuroprotective genes, they also upregulate immune response genes, likely of glial origin, that may cause tissue damage and apoptosis. Microarray gene expression studies on steroid-induced glaucoma have shown that steroids induce dose dependent, differential gene profiles in human trabecular meshwork (TM) cells [23-26]. Currently, the TM epithelium is considered to be the target tissue and the myocilin gene, which is expressed mainly in TM, the top candidate gene for the development of steroid-induced glaucoma. The myocilin protein clogs the TM that causes increased intraocular pressure (IOP) [27]. Although an elevated IOP is a significant risk factor for the development of glaucoma, it is important to note that sight-threatening effects of glaucoma are not necessarily coming from increased IOP but from retinal and optic nerve neurodegeneration.

We did genomics expression analysis of Dex and TAA intravitreal injections in the mouse retinas at clinically relevant time points of 1 week and 1 month. More than 1500 genes were found to be differentially expressed at the level of 99% statistical significance. Furthermore, statistical analysis for each of the time points separately identified groups of genes that are common and similarly regulated for both steroids as well as a set of unique genes differentially regulated by each steroid. [28]. For example, in week 1 postinjection, common upregulated genes for both dexamethasone and triamcinolone were stress response proteins and genes with a role in immune response and apoptosis, members of TGFβ receptor signaling and TNFα signaling cascade, as well as Semaphorin signaling, which VEGF signaling is part of. Besides the common ones, dexamethasone uniquely activated retinal glia macrophages and genes that are regulated by NFkappaB and p53, while triamcinolone's week 1 targets were primarily genes from the folate pathway and dopamine metabolism. Pathway analysis demonstrated that some of the biological pathways activated are unique for each steroid, although even in the pathways that are common, different set of genes might be affected differently by different steroid. For example, both dexamethasone and triamcinolone activated Semaphorin signaling pathway, but one week after dexamethasone treatment we observed upregulation of ligands Sema3, Sema4, and Sema5a, on the glial side, and Plexins A and A2 receptors on the neuronal side. One week after TAA injection we observed upregulation of Sema4 and Sema3, while

Plexins A and A2 were downregulated. Our results, and results of several other investigators [23-26, 29], demonstrate that each steroid has discrete specificity both clinically and biologically. Small differences in the structure can result in targeting different sets of genes, or different biological pathways. We will discuss the significance of these observations a bit later.

Several of the genes we identified upregulated by dexamethasone are identical or related to the genes identified by microarray analysis of DBA/J mouse, a mouse glaucoma model [30, 31]. Although, it still remains to be seen whether upregulation of these genes have a protective or damaging effect on retinal and optic nerve degeneration as well as glaucoma development.

One of the top pathways identified was 'Semaphorin Signaling in Neurons'. Semaphorins are signaling molecules that act as neuronal as well as vascular growth guidance molecules. Disregulation of this pathway can lead to inhibition and/or apoptosis of neuronal tissue, as well as disregulated growth of vascular tissue. In addition to their role in axonal guidance, semaphorins also have a major role in immune response. At one week after dexamethasone treatment we observed upregulation of several of Sema ligands (Sema3, Sema4, and Sema5a) expressed on glial cells, and their Plexin receptors (A and A2), expressed on the neuronal side. Semaphorin 4A has an important role in the visual system development, and Sema4A mouse knockout develops severe retinal degeneration [32]. Sema3A has been found to be secreted by ischemic neurons in the avascular retina in the response to the pro-inflammatory cytokine IL-1beta, thus preventing vascular regeneration in proliferative retinopathies [33]. The role of Sema3E in eye therapy is still being worked out: both inhibition of Sema3E protein [34] as well as intravitreal application [35] are being considered for therapeutic anti-angiogenesis. Sema5A, upregulated one week after dexamethasone injection, has been shown to promote angiogenesis by increasing endothelial cell proliferation, migration, and decreasing apoptosis in vitro [36].

There was upregulation of somatostatin receptor Sstr2 1 week post injection. Somatostatin signaling regulates glutamate release in the retina [37], and it has been suggested that Sstr2 has an anti-angiogenic role in retina [38] therefore its upregulation of Sstr2, might be a result of the protective effect of dexamethasone against inflammation.

At one month post-injection of dexamethasone we observed upregulation Aryl-hydrocarbon receptor (AhR). It has been shown that Ahr has a regulatory role for small heat shock proteins induced in retina and other tissues of the eye [39]. Several human retinal dystrophies such as Leber congenital amaurosis, juvenile retinitis pigmentosa and dominant cone-rod dystrophy are mapped to AhR pathway [40, 41].

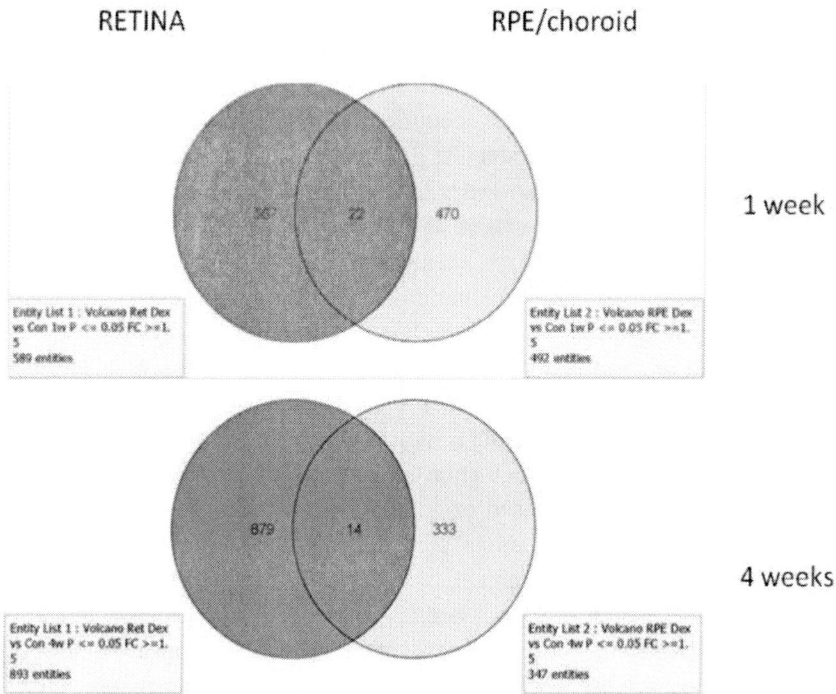

Figure 3. Tissue specific differences in the gene expression in response to intravitreal dexamethasone application in the mouse eye.

Members of the AhR family play critical roles in a broad range of biological functions including regulation of circadian rhythm, neurogenesis, hypoxia response and drug metabolism.

Our focus in data interpretation was on genes with known neuroprotective vs. neurodegenerative effects and/or known role in ophthalmic or neurodegenerative diseases. We have identified several genes and pathways that appear to be affected by intravitreal dexamethasone injections. Perhaps modulation of some of these potential targets in combination with steroid intravitreal therapy will in the future lead to reduced side-effects.

When we examined gene expression profile of the RPE at the same time points (unpublished data), we found strong tissue specific expression and response to intravitreal dexamethasone application. Figure 3 illustrates dramatic differences between these two tissue types.

Immune Response Regulation by Dexamethasone and Implications for Treatment of Retinal Disease

Glucocorticoids can regulate inflammatory and autoimmune response by directly suppressing innate and cellular immune response. There are two main types of cellular immune response – Th1 being cell-mediated, while Th2 is humoral-mediated immunity. Some of the typical cytokines that represent mediators of these actions are IL-12 for Th1, IL-4 for Th2 and IL-17 for Th17. Franchimont et al have shown that dexamethasone selectively inhibits IL-12 inducible IFN-gamma secretion and Stat4 phosphorylation, in both NK and T-cells, without altering IL-4 phosphorylation. This might be one of the mechanisms by which dexamethasone shift immune response from cellular (Th1) to humoral (Th2) [42]. One of the early relevant finding for eye research was that repeated pre-treatment with dexamethasone was able to suppress early and late phase of topically induced ocular anaphylaxis in rats [43].

Relatively recently, a novel type of Th cells has been described, and its importance is steadily growing – Th17, T-cells which selectively produces pro-inflammatory cytokines, such as IL-17, IL-21 and IL-22. Th17 cells are now known to play an important role in the pathogenesis of inflammation and autoimmune diseases [44]. Figure 4 illustrates these three branches of immune system and their interaction.

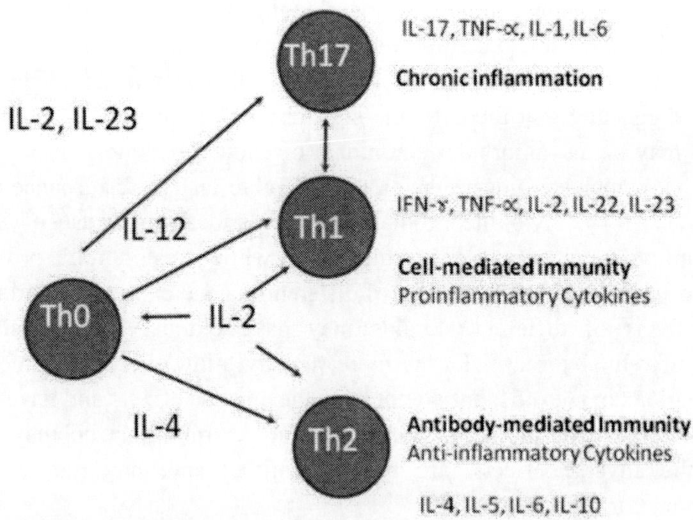

Figure 4. The schematics of the Th1, Th2 and Th17 branches of immune system and their interactions.

Table 1. Retinal diseases have differential disregulations of Th1/Th2/Th17 branches of immune system

Retinal Diseases	Th1 (IL-1, IL-2)	Th2 (IL-4, IL-6, IL-10)	Th17 (IL-17, IL-22)
CME		+ [52]	
DME	+ [53]	++ [49, 53]	
RVO		++ [49, 54, 55]	+ [55]
AMD	+ [56]	++ [56]	+ [57]

In addition to cytokines, induction of TGFbeta-1 and retinoic acid-related orphan receptor-gammat (RORgammat) lead to differentiation of Th-17 cells in mice. Role of dexamethasone is still controversial. There is report that dexamethasone can inhibit the release of IL-17 likely by inhibiting RORgammat expression and blocking Th17 differentiation in asthmatic Balb/c mice [45]. On the other hand, in a model of chronic allergic airway inflammation in Th17-deficient mice in T cells, where Th-17 cells induce airway remodeling independent of Th2 response, Zhao et al. showed that dexamethasone inhibited eosinophilia, present in acute inflammation, but not neutrophilia, hallmark of chronic disease, and enhanced Th17 development in vitro [46].

Our results suggests that there may be a preference between steroids as to which branch of immune system they act upon, as well as tissue specificity (Smit-McBride et al, manuscript in submission). The main branches of the immune system are represented on the Figure 4. The clinical evidence is mounting suggesting that the cytokine signaling produced by CD4+ T helper (Th) cells may be an important determinant of clinical pathology in a variety of diseases in which steroids are being tested (Table 1). The disturbance of the balance of Th1/Th2 cytokine production is an underlying cause of neural damage in several neurologic diseases, while restoration promotes neuroprotection [47-51]. The finding of differential gene expression and tissue specific effects of different steroids may have clinical implications for treatment of retinal disease. Furthermore, it may allow the development of new generations of steroids that do not have the adverse effects and have more specific targeting. Additionally, biomarkers for determining who may be at risk for the adverse effects, are being identified and may reduce these complications for future use.

Clinical Usage of Dexamethasone

Popular Formulations of Dexamethasone

Although there are several steroid formulations that may be used, this article focuses on the use of intravitreal dexamethasone. Dexamethasone is a potent anti-inflammatory agent that inhibits multiple inflammatory cytokines. Dexamethasone has a relatively short half-life (3.5 hours), but is 5 times more potent than other steroid formulations, including intravitreal triamcinolone. Intravitreal dexamethasone comes in a 4mg/ml solution, and may be injected in the vitreous space at a dosage of 0.4 mg.

Despite the anti-inflammatory benefits of dexamethasone, the short half-life of 3 hours limits the clinical use. This limitation is addressed via a biodegradable dexamethasone implant—Ozurdex (DEX implant, Allergan, Inc., Irvine, CA). Ozurdex delivers an extended release of dexamethasone via an intravitreal injection to modulate various macular and retinal disorders. The implant is made of a solid polymer (Novadur™, Allergan, Irvine, CA, USA), that initially releases a burst of dexamethasone to achieve a therapeutic concentration followed by a lower sustained release of the drug. Ozurdex allows a longer duration of pharmacological effect with lower administration frequency compared to other intravitreal steroids. The benefits of Ozurdex may last up to 6 months in the eye, but clinicians often report a shorter duration of action. It should be noted that the FDA has approved the use of intraocular steroids only for a select number of conditions [1]. Ozurdex was approved as first line therapy for macular edema secondary to vein occlusions in 2009, and for treatment of non-infectious uveitis in 2010 [58]. However, retinal clinicians often use Ozurdex "off label" to treat a wider range of ocular disorders, namely macular edema from diabetic retinopathy or post-surgical cystoid macular edema.

Clinically Usage of Steroids Based on Disease

Endophthalmitis

Intraocular dexamethasone was first used in the 1970s to reduce the inflammatory response in the treatment of bacterial endophthalmitis in conjunction with antibiotic therapy. Endophthalmitis is a severe inflammation of the eye secondary to contaminating microorganisms introduced during surgery, penetrating trauma, or endogenous spread. Despite appropriate therapeutic intervention, bacterial endophthalmitis frequently results in visual loss, and potentially loss of the eye. The first line of therapy remains intravitreal antibiotics or vitrectomy surgery (EVS study [97]); however, dexamethasone is often added as an adjunct to the antibiotic regimen based on its rapid mechanism of action for modulating the inflammatory response. Currently, intravitreal dexamethasone's role in combating the destructive inflammatory response in endophthalmitis remains controversial, as the literature provides conflicting results. In 1974 Graham and Peyman described the beneficial addition of intravitreal dexamethasone to antibiotic therapy in the rabbit model for reduction of the inflammatory response in the anterior and posterior chambers, vitreous, retina, and choroid [59]. Intravitreal dexamethasone has been used as an adjunct to intravitreal antibiotics in the management of bacterial endophthalmitis—namely in cases with gram-negative endophthalmitis [60]. In the rabbit model, Streptococcus pneumonia infected eyes treated with vancomycin and dexamethasone had significantly less intraocular inflammation and more preservation of retinal tissue than untreated eyes or eyes treated with vancomycin alone [61]. Clinically, several authors showed favorable visual results when dexamethasone was used in the treatment of post-cataract endophthalmitis [62, 63]. A recent study demonstrated that intravitreal dexamethasone improved vision without prolonging infection in patients with bleb-induced endophthalmitis, a particularly severe form of endophthalmitis [64]. However, other studies have shown no difference in the visual acuity of eyes treated with and without dexamethasone [65] and some studies have even shown negative visual results [66]. In 2004, 43% of retina specialists reported that they use intravitreal dexamethasone in conjunction with intraocular antibiotics to treat postsurgical endophthalmitis [67].

Trauma

Intraocular steroids have also been used to modulate the inflammatory response in surgical and nonsurgical trauma. The ultimate success rate of vitreoretinal surgery is limited by development of proliferative vitreoretinopathy (PVR). Stages of vitreoretinal scarring include cellular activation, proliferation, extracellular matrix elaboration and remodeling, and contraction [68]. Anti-inflammatory agents such as dexamethasone and other corticosteroids have been used to limit the process of vitreo-retinal scarring. A single intravitreal injection of 1 mg of dexamethasone has shown to reduce the rate of development of tractional retinal detachment and retinal neovascularization in rabbits after injection of homologous fibroblasts. [69]. Subconjunctival dexamethasone injection at the conclusion of intraocular surgery and frequent topical corticosteroid treatment are commonly used techniques for prophylaxis against postoperative inflammation and fibrin formation [68]. However, intravitreal dexamethasone (0.8 mg) at the end of vitrectomy for complicated diabetic retinopathy did not successfully reduce intraocular inflammation, flare, or fibrin formation [70]. Another study by Chalam et al showed that patients who received 0.4mg of intravitreal dexamethasone at the end of vitrectomy surgery for proliferative diabetic retinopathy or macular puckers showed significant reduction in postoperative inflammation as measured by aqueous cell and flare intensity on postoperative day 1, 10, and 90 [71].

Exudative Macular Degeneration

Intravitreal dexamethasone is also used in clinical practice as a part of adjuvant therapy to treat wet macular degeneration. Wet macular degeneration, a potentially blinding ocular condition, is a multi-factorial condition that involves neovascularization, vascular leakage, and inflammation. A triple therapy approach to wet macular degeneration that addresses these pathologies can be employed when more traditional methods (i.e. repeated anti-VEGF agents) have failed. Triple therapy consists of reduced-fluence photodynamic therapy, an anti-VEGF agent, and dexamethasone. The range of dexamethasone dose used ranges from 200-800 micrograms per injection. Several recent studies [72-74] have shown that triple therapy may reduce the total number of injections needed in some patients and stabilize vision in those patients who do not respond to single therapy with anti-VEGF agents. A recent study demonstrated that the combination of intravitreal anti-VEGF with dexamethasone and full-fluence photodynamic therapy provided visual and anatomic improvement and a good safety profile [75]. Patients who received triple-therapy required a lower number of total injections and a longer interval of time before repeat injections were necessary. Of note, no adverse effects of intravitreal dexamethasone were observed in the mean follow up period of 14 months. A study investigating quadruple therapy for macular degeneration (low-fluence PDT, followed 24 h later by a 0.4-ml core pars plana vitrectomy with intravitreal injection of 0.8 mg dexamethasone and 1.25 mg bevacizumab) showed sustained visual improvement over 14 months, without any adverse side-effects of dexamethasone [76]. Although the standard treatment of wet macular degeneration remains monthly anti-VEGF injections, intravitreal dexamethasone may be an important adjuvant treatment for some patients.

Diabetic Macular Edema

Diabetic macular edema is a visually-threatening eye disorder that is often a challenge to treat. Thermal laser photocoagulation remains the only FDA approved treatment for diabetic macular edema. However, thermal laser is not an ideal treatment option for patients who have vascular leakage within the foveal-avascular zone, who have a significant amount of macular edema, or who have had an inadequate response to past laser therapy. Although the FDA has not approved the use of Ozurdex for the treatment of diabetic macular edema, it is increasingly becoming a popular therapeutic option, especially in post-vitrectomized eyes [77]. Increased production of inflammatory mediators and vascular permeability factors contribute to diabetic macular edema, and these processes are stabilized by corticosteroids [78]. Several studies have shown Ozurdex's benefit at reducing macular edema and vascular leakage [77, 78]. One study found that the dexamethasone implant improved visual acuity for up to 6 months in patients with macular edema due to a variety of causes including diabetic retinopathy [79]. In a subgroup analysis of 171 eyes with persistent diabetic macular edema, the dexamethasone implant resulted in improvement in best corrected visual acuity at three months, but this was lost after 180 days - and steroid treatment groups had an increased incidence of elevated IOP [80]. A study in patients' who were status post vitrectomy showed that a dexamethasone implant resulted in statistically and clinically significant improvements in both vision and vascular leakage from diabetic macular edema, with an acceptable safety profile [77]. It is important to note, however, that the benefit of intravitreal dexamethasone tapered from week 1 to week 26 of the study.

Retinal Vein Occlusion

Retinal vein occlusion is second to diabetic retinopathy as a cause of vision loss from an underlying retinal vascular disorder. Retinal vein occlusion leads to vision loss from macular edema and ocular ischemia. The FDA approved the use of Ozurdex in the treatment of vein occlusions based on two identical, multicenter, masked, randomized, 6-month, sham-controlled clinical trials that included 1267 patients with vision loss from BRVO or CRVO [80]. Haller et al. showed the safety and efficacy of the dexamethasone intravitreal implant compared with sham control. Improvement in mean best corrected visual acuity was greater in the DEX implant groups compared with sham at all follow-up visits (P< or =0.006) over 6 months. The dexamethasone implant reduced the risk of vision loss and improved the speed and incidence of visual improvement in eyes with macular edema secondary to BRVO or CRVO. Further, the incidence of DEX implant-treated eyes with IOP of > or =25 was not different from sham by day 180, and there were no patients that required cataract surgery at 6 months.

Haller et al. then extended the study design for 6 more months (in an open-label extension of the study) [80]. She reported that out of the 1256 patients included in the study-extension, 997 patients required a second treatment of Ozurdex implant based on decreased visual acuity or increase in macular thickness at day 180. Over the 12 month study period, patients who received either a single or repeat treatment of DEX implant had improved visual acuity and decrease in macular edema compared to sham. The rates of complications between the groups that received one implant injection versus two implant injections were similar, except the group that received two injections had a higher rate of cataract formation at the end of study period (29.8% versus 5.7%). Other recent studies have also demonstrated the safety and efficacy of the Ozurdex implant in treatment of vein occlusions [80-82].

In our experience, we have found dramatic improvements in macular edema in patients with retinal vein occlusions. For example, in our practice we saw a 64 year old male with a history of a vein occlusion with significant macular edema with count finger vision that did not improve with 5 prior intravitreal anti-VEGF injections (Figure 5). He received an Ozurdex injection, and two months after the injection he experienced a significant decrease in macular edema and improvement in vision to 20/200 (Figure 6). At the two month follow up, he did not have an elevated intraocular pressure.

Although Ozurdex is the first FDA approved pharmacologic treatment for vein occlusions, work still needs to be done to determine the best frequency of drug administration. Haller et al. demonstrated effectively of Ozurdex implant with either one or two intravitreal injections over a 12 month period. Qureques et al. demonstrated that repeated intravitreal Ozurdex on a "per-needed' basis (with a retreatment interval <6 months) had benefits in the treatment of ME due to RVO [81]. Matonti et al. reported a case of a 75 year old female who benefited from a series of four Ozurdex injections over 17 months [83]. Although Ozurdex remains the only FDA approved treatment of macular edema from central retina vein occlusions, it is interesting that in a recent 2012 Membership Survey of Preferences and Trends by the American Society of Retinal Specialists, 36% of US/Canadian members and 50% of international members reported not having experience with use of the drug. Interestingly, about a quarter of all members in the survey reported that Ozurdex is more effective than Triamcinolone in treating central retinal vein occlusions.

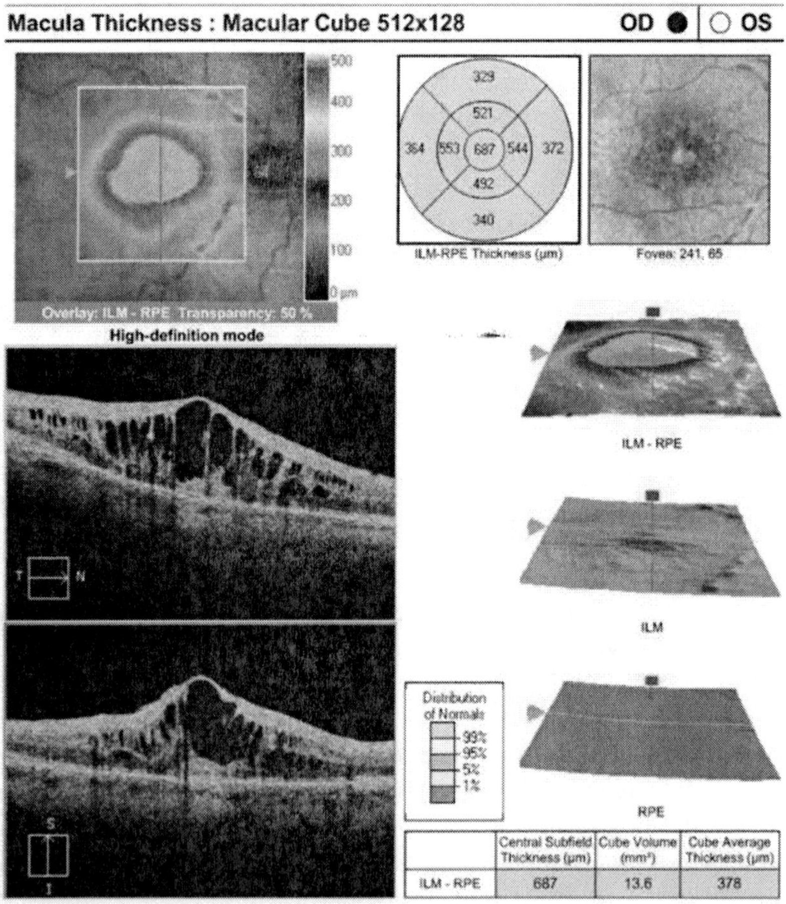

Figure 5. Optical coherence tomography (OCT) image of macula in patient with cystoid macular edema from a retina vein occlusion.

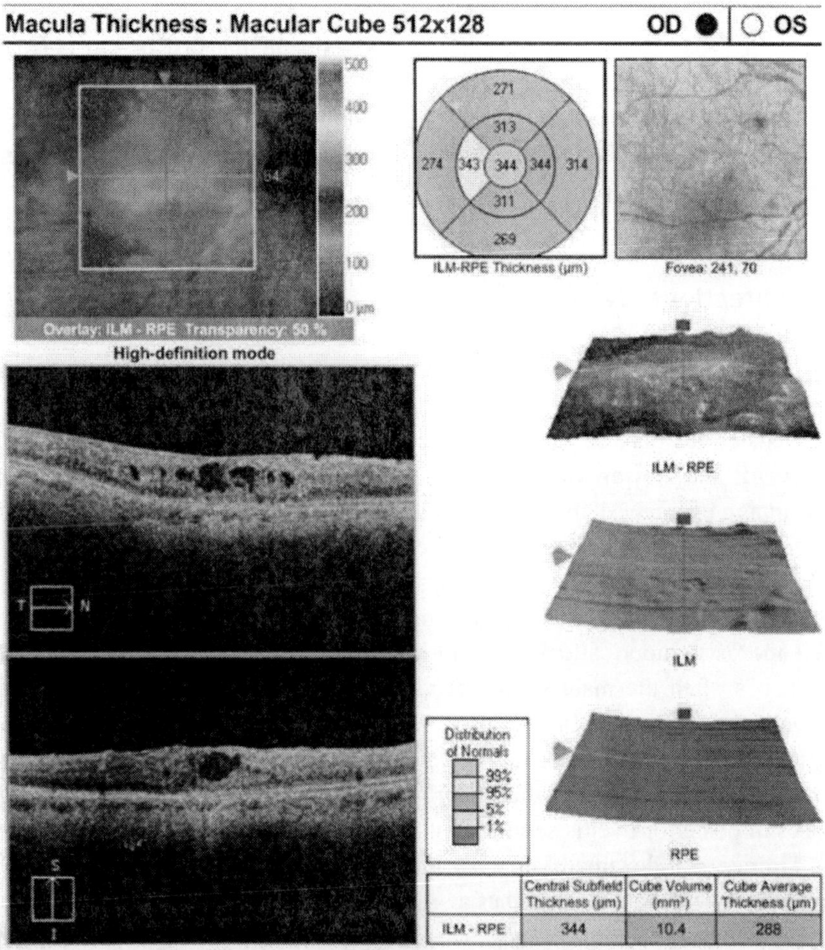

Figure 6. OCT image of patient in Figure 5, 2 months after intravitreal injection of Ozurdex steroid implant.

Pseudophakic Cystoid Macular Edema

Despite advances in modern cataract surgery, pseudophakic cystoids macular edema (PCME) remains a common problem that may cause vision loss during the post-operative period. Several treatment options are available, but most clinicians use a step-wise treatment approach that starts with topical medical treatment (topical NSAIDS and steroids) and may progress to surgical intervention, namely pars plana vitrectomy. In cases of severe or refractory cystoids macular edema, subtenon's or intravitreal steroids are commonly employed [84]. Some clinicians use steroid implants the first-line of treatment in PCME [85]. The Ozurdex implant would have a role in treating PCME, especially in vitrectomized eyes. Unfortunately, to our knowledge, there are no published randomized clinical trials to compare intravitreal dexamethasone to other established treatment modalities [86].

Noninfectious Uveitis

Uveitis is responsible for 30,000 new cases of legal blindness annually in the Western world [87]. Topical, systemic, periocular, and intravitreal corticosteroids play an important role in the treatment of noninfectious forms of uveitis and they are the first-line treatments in this condition. They offer the advantage of direct delivery to the site of inflammation while minimizing and avoiding a host of systemic side effects seen with oral and intravenous administration of corticosteroids. Systemic steroids are associated with fluid retention, hypertension, hyperglycemia, greater susceptibility to infections, osteoporosis, mood alteration, and psychosis. In posterior uveitis macular edema is often the main source of vision loss. Intravitreal treatment directly targets this site and may be used as monotherapy or in conjunction with systemic immunosuppression depending on the absence or presence of extraocular manifestation the underlying auto immune condition. In chronic cases of posterior uveitis serial intravitreal treatments may be necessary.

Intravitreal dexamethasone has the advantage of office-based implantation procedure with topical anesthesia. A 26-week trial was performed studying single treatment with 0.7-mg DEX implant and 0.35-mg DEX implant compared to a control sham group [88]. Proportion of eyes with a vitreous haze score of zero at week 8 was 47% with the 0.7-mg DEX implant, 35% with the 0.35% DEX implant, and 12% with the sham groups. At all time points, the proportion of eyes with improvement in vitreous haze was greater in the dexamethasone treated groups, seen in over 90% by 6 weeks compared with 46% of sham-treated eyes. Less than 10% of eyes receiving the 700 μg implant had an intraocular pressure rise of over 25 mm Hg at any point, and no patient had progression of cataracts. In a comparison based series, Arcinue et al evaluated the efficacy and safety of the flucinolone acetonide (Retisert) implant compared with the dexamethasone (Ozurdex) implant in 27 eyes that noninfectious uveitis [89]. Of note, Ozurdex is implanted in the eye in the office-setting, but the Retisert implant requires surgical intervention in the operating room with sedation. No significant differences were seen in terms of improvement in inflammatory score and best-corrected visual acuity (BCVA) in both groups. Eyes with the Ozurdex were 5 times more likely to receive a second implant compared to Retisert (P=0.02). No eyes in the Ozurdex group needed additional glaucoma medications, surgery, or laser compared to 44% of eyes in the Retisert group.

Toxoplasmosis

Kishore and Peyman in 2001 described a new method of management of toxoplasmic retinochoroiditis by using intravitreal injections of clindamycin (1mg/0.1ml) and dexamethasone (1mg/0.1ml) [90]. A lower dose of intravitreal dexamethasone (0.4 mg/0.1 ml) in combination with a higher dose of clindamycin (1.5 mg/0.1 ml) has also shown to be effective for treatment of zone 1 toxoplasmic retinochoroiditis in cases of intolerance to oral medication, contraindication to oral medication secondary to pregnancy, and lack of response and progression of disease despite oral antimicrobial and anti-inflammatory treatment [91].

Complications

Chronic administration of steroids can have systemic and local side effects. Topical, periocular, and intravitreal treatment of ocular disorders limits the systemic side effects and there is minimal systemic absorption following local administration of steroids [1]. However, the risk of local side effects such as cataract formation, increased intraocular pressure, and development of glaucoma may not be avoided [92]. Each technique for delivery of corticosteroid to the eye may also present its own inherent risks. Periocular steroid treatment carries a risk of inadvertent globe penetration, extraocular muscle injury, ptosis, and local skin depigmentation [87]. The risks of intravitreal injection include endophthalmitis, retinal detachment, vitreous hemorrhage, and the risk of cataract formation and IOP elevation is higher with intravitreal administration of corticosteroids.

Despite the known benefits of reducing inflammation in several macular diseases, intravitreal glucocorticoids may lead to progression of cataracts and development of steroid-induced glaucoma that are unique to this drug-class. Studies on steroid-induced glaucoma have shown that corticosteroids induce dose-dependent, differential gene profiles in human trabecular meshwork cells, revealed by microarray technology [23, 25]. Microarray analysis has also shown that intravitreal corticosteroids may upregulate immune response genes, likely in glial cells that may cause damage to retinal neural tissue [28].

In the landmark Haller et al. study the percentage of DEX implant-treated eyes with IOP of > or =25 mmHg peaked at 16% at 60 days in the Dex-treated group, but there was no difference from the sham control group at day 180 [93]. Statistically significant side effects of the dexamethasone treated group not found in the sham group also included eye pain and anterior chamber cells. It is important to note that although there were no significant differences between the rate of cataract formation between the treated and the sham control group, the study length was only 6 months. In Haller et al.'s extension follow up of 12 months [94], cataract progression occurred in 90 of 302 phakic eyes (29.8%) that received 2 DEX implant 0.7 mg injections versus 5 of 88 sham-treated phakic eyes (5.7%). At 12 months, 10.3% of patients who received two dexamethasone injections required IOP-lowering medications. When using Ozurdex for uveitis patients, the incidence of cataract progression reported was 15% with the 0.7-mg DEX implant, 12% with the 0.35-mg DEX implant, and 7% of the sham control group (P>0.05). Throughout the 26 week study, the percentage of eyes in the 0.7mg DEX implant group requiring IOP lowering medication was 23% and no eyes required incisional surgery as intervention for elevated IOP.

Some unique complications have been reported using the DEX implant as compared to the DEX solution. Reports of anterior dislocation of the DEX implant have been noted. In some cases repositioning has been successful by dilation of the eye and placement of patient in supine reclined position [95]. The risk of anterior chamber migration of the DEX implant is increased in cases of prior vitrectomy with prone positioning of patient in dilated state. Iris claw lenses and zonular rupture increase the risk of this complication, and in patients without integrity of the zonules and the posterior capsule there is a potential risk of anterior chamber migration of the DEX implant [96].

Conclusion

1. Dexamethasone has tissue-specific effects on gene expression in retina and RPE tissue.

2. Dexamethasone has different effects on tissues whose effects are modulated by different glucocorticoid receptor interactions. The biological effects of steroids are then mediated through several mechanisms involving, genomic and non-genomic effects with subsequent transactivation or transrepression. Lastly, epigenetic effects of steroids are emerging as important determinants of action.
3. Dexamethasone clinically has a short half-life, but is highly potent. The biodegradable implant Ozurdex, allows for sustainable delivery in the vitreous and lasts 4-6 months.
4. Dexamethasone affects clinically relevant pathways involving inflammation, proliferation, apoptosis, and oxidative stress.
5. The primary clinical side effects of dexamethasone use include cataracts formation and glaucoma.
6. Dexamethasone has clinically been used to treat cystoid macular degeneration from surgery, retinal vein occlusion, exudative age-related macular degeneration and diabetes. Other uses include treatment of non-infectious uveitis.
7. Ozurdex has been FDA approved for the treatment of retinal vein occlusions and non-infectious uveitis. Ongoing studies are exploring the possible usefulness of Ozurdex in the treatment of diabetic macular edema.

References

[1] Kiernan, D. F. and W. F. Mieler, The use of intraocular corticosteroids. *Expert Opin. Pharmacother.*, 2009. 10(15): p. 2511-25.

[2] Scott, I. U., et al., A randomized trial comparing the efficacy and safety of intravitreal triamcinolone with standard care to treat vision loss associated with macular Edema secondary to branch retinal vein occlusion: the Standard Care vs Corticosteroid for Retinal Vein Occlusion (SCORE) study report 6. *Arch. Ophthalmol.*, 2009. 127(9): p. 1115-28.

[3] Rhen, T. and J. A. Cidlowski, Antiinflammatory action of gluco-corticoids--new mechanisms for old drugs. *N. Engl. J. Med.*, 2005. 353(16): p. 1711-23.

[4] Laudet, V., et al., Evolution of the nuclear receptor gene superfamily. *EMBO J.*, 1992. 11(3): p. 1003-13.

[5] Biddie, S. C. and G. L. Hager, Glucocorticoid receptor dynamics and gene regulation. *Stress*, 2009. 12(3): p. 193-205.

[6] Stolte, E. H., et al., Evolution of glucocorticoid receptors with different glucocorticoid sensitivity. *J. Endocrinol.*, 2006. 190(1): p. 17-28.

[7] Yudt, M. R., et al., Molecular origins for the dominant negative function of human glucocorticoid receptor beta. *Mol. Cell Biol.*, 2003. 23(12): p. 4319-30.

[8] Lu, N. Z. and J. A. Cidlowski, The origin and functions of multiple human glucocorticoid receptor isoforms. *Ann. N. Y. Acad. Sci.*, 2004. 1024: p. 102-23.

[9] McKay, L. I. and J. A. Cidlowski, Molecular control of immune/inflammatory responses: interactions between nuclear factor-kappa B and steroid receptor-signaling pathways. *Endocr. Rev.*, 1999. 20(4): p. 435-59.

[10] McKay, L. I. and J. A. Cidlowski, Cross-talk between nuclear factor-kappa B and the steroid hormone receptors: mechanisms of mutual antagonism. *Mol. Endocrinol.*, 1998. 12(1): p. 45-56.

[11] Barnes, P. J., Anti-inflammatory actions of glucocorticoids: molecular mechanisms. *Clin. Sci.* (Lond), 1998. 94(6): p. 557-72.

[12] Barnes, P. J., Corticosteroid effects on cell signalling. *Eur. Respir. J.*, 2006. 27(2): p. 413-26.

[13] Barnes, P. J., Corticosteroids: the drugs to beat. *Eur. J. Pharmacol.*, 2006. 533(1-3): p. 2-14.

[14] Glotin, A. L., et al., Sustained versus transient ERK1/2 signaling underlies the anti- and proapoptotic effects of oxidative stress in human RPE cells. *Invest. Ophthalmol. Vis. Sci.*, 2006. 47(10): p. 4614-23.

[15] Hafezi-Moghadam, A., et al., Acute cardiovascular protective effects of corticosteroids are mediated by non-transcriptional activation of endothelial nitric oxide synthase. *Nat. Med.*, 2002. 8(5): p. 473-9.

[16] Cato, A. C., A. Nestl, and S. Mink, Rapid actions of steroid receptors in cellular signaling pathways. Sci. STKE, 2002. 2002(138): p. re9.

[17] Wan, E. S., et al., Systemic steroid exposure is associated with differential methylation in chronic obstructive pulmonary disease. *Am. J. Respir. Crit. Care Med.*, 2012. 186(12): p. 1248-55.

[18] Crudo, A., et al., Glucocorticoid programming of the fetal male hippocampal epigenome. *Endocrinology*, 2013. 154(3): p. 1168-80.

[19] McMaster, A. and D. W. Ray, Modelling the glucocorticoid receptor and producing therapeutic agents with anti-inflammatory effects but reduced side-effects. *Exp. Physiol.*, 2007. 92(2): p. 299-309.

[20] Ray, D. W., et al., Structure/function of the human glucocorticoid receptor: tyrosine 735 is important for transactivation. *Mol. Endocrinol.*, 1999. 13(11): p. 1855-63.

[21] Kauppi, B., et al., The three-dimensional structures of antagonistic and agonistic forms of the glucocorticoid receptor ligand-binding domain: RU-486 induces a transconformation that leads to active antagonism. *J. Biol. Chem.*, 2003. 278(25): p. 22748-54.

[22] Garside, H., et al., Glucocorticoid ligands specify different interactions with NF-kappaB by allosteric effects on the glucocorticoid receptor DNA binding domain. *J. Biol. Chem.*, 2004. 279(48): p. 50050-9.

[23] Fan, B. J., et al., Gene expression profiles of human trabecular meshwork cells induced by triamcinolone and dexamethasone. *Invest. Ophthalmol. Vis. Sci.*, 2008. 49(5): p. 1886-97.

[24] Diskin, S., et al., Detection of differentially expressed glycogenes in trabecular meshwork of eyes with primary open-angle glaucoma. *Invest. Ophthalmol. Vis. Sci.*, 2006. 47(4): p. 1491-9.

[25] Rozsa, F. W., et al., Gene expression profile of human trabecular meshwork cells in response to long-term dexamethasone exposure. *Mol. Vis.*, 2006. 12: p. 125-41.

[26] Nehme, A., et al., Glucocorticoids with different chemical structures but similar glucocorticoid receptor potency regulate subsets of common and unique genes in human trabecular meshwork cells. *BMC Med. Genomics*, 2009. 2: p. 58.

[27] Paper, W., et al., Elevated amounts of myocilin in the aqueous humor of transgenic mice cause significant changes in ocular gene expression. *Exp. Eye Res.,* 2008. 87(3): p. 257-67.

[28] Smit-McBride, Z., et al., In vivo gene expression profiling of retina postintravitreal injections of dexamethasone and triamcinolone at clinically relevant time points for patient care. *Invest. Ophthalmol. Vis. Sci.*, 2011. 52(12): p. 8965-78.

[29] Edelman, J. L., Differentiating intraocular glucocorticoids. *Ophthalmologica*, 2010. 224 Suppl 1: p. 25-30.

[30] Steele, M. R., et al., Microarray analysis of retinal gene expression in the DBA/2J model of glaucoma. *Invest. Ophthalmol. Vis. Sci.*, 2006. 47(3): p. 977-85.

[31] Fan, W., et al., Early Involvement of Immune/Inflammatory Response Genes in Retinal Degeneration in DBA/2J Mice. *Ophthalmol. Eye Dis.*, 2010. 1: p. 23-41.

[32] Rice, D. S., et al., Severe retinal degeneration associated with disruption of semaphorin 4A. *Invest. Ophthalmol. Vis. Sci.*, 2004. 45(8): p. 2767-77.

[33] Joyal, J. S., et al., Ischemic neurons prevent vascular regeneration of neural tissue by secreting semaphorin 3A. *Blood*, 2011.

[34] Moriya, J., et al., Inhibition of semaphorin as a novel strategy for therapeutic angiogenesis. *Circ. Res.*, 2010. 106(2): p. 391-8.

[35] Fukushima, Y., et al., Sema3E-PlexinD1 signaling selectively suppresses disoriented angiogenesis in ischemic retinopathy in mice. *J. Clin. Invest.*, 2011. 121(5): p. 1974-85.

[36] Sadanandam, A., et al., Semaphorin 5A promotes angiogenesis by increasing endothelial cell proliferation, migration, and decreasing apoptosis. *Microvasc. Res.*, 2010. 79(1): p. 1-9.

[37] Dal Monte, M., et al., Somatostatin inhibits potassium-evoked glutamate release by activation of the sst(2) somatostatin receptor in the mouse retina. *Naunyn Schmiedebergs Arch. Pharmacol.*, 2003. 367(2): p. 188-92.

[38] Dal Monte, M., et al., Antiangiogenic role of somatostatin receptor 2 in a model of hypoxia-induced neovascularization in the retina: results from transgenic mice. *Invest. Ophthalmol. Vis. Sci.*, 2007. 48(8): p. 3480-9.

[39] Liu, S. and J. Piatigorsky, Regulation of Mouse Small Heat Shock Protein alphab-Crystallin Gene by Aryl Hydrocarbon Receptor. *PLoS One,* 2011. 6(4): p. e17904.

[40] Jacobson, S. G., et al., Human retinal disease from AIPL1 gene mutations: foveal cone loss with minimal macular photoreceptors and rod function remaining. *Invest. Ophthalmol. Vis. Sci.*, 2011. 52(1): p. 70-9.

[41] Perrault, I., et al., Leber congenital amaurosis. *Mol. Genet. Metab.*, 1999. 68(2): p. 200-8.

[42] Franchimont, D., et al., Inhibition of Th1 immune response by glucocorticoids: dexamethasone selectively inhibits IL-12-induced Stat4 phosphorylation in T lymphocytes. *J. Immunol.*, 2000. 164(4): p. 1768-74.

[43] Trocme, S. D., et al., Effects of topical pre-treatment with dexamethasone on the immediate and late phases of topically induced ocular anaphylaxis in the rat. *Acta Ophthalmol.* (Copenh), 1988. 66(1): p. 24-32.

[44] Takatori, H., et al., New complexities in helper T cell fate determination and the implications for autoimmune diseases. *Mod. Rheumatol.*, 2008. 18(6): p. 533-41.

[45] Hu, S. M., et al., [Effects of dexamethasone on intracellular expression of Th17 cytokine interleukin 17 in asthmatic mice]. Nan Fang Yi Ke Da Xue Xue Bao, 2009. 29(6): p. 1185-8.

[46] Zhao, J., C. M. Lloyd, and A. Noble, Th17 responses in chronic allergic airway inflammation abrogate regulatory T-cell-mediated tolerance and contribute to airway remodeling. *Mucosal Immunol.*, 2013. 6(2): p. 335-46.

[47] Huang, P., S. S. Zhang, and C. Zhang, Erratum: The two sides of cytokine signaling and glaucomatous optic neuropathy. *J. Ocul. Biol. Dis. Infor.*, 2009. 2(3): p. 98-103.

[48] Huang, P., S. S. Zhang, and C. Zhang, The two sides of cytokine signaling and glaucomatous optic neuropathy. *J. Ocul. Biol. Dis. Infor.*, 2009. 2(2): p. 78-83.

[49] Yoshimura, T., et al., Comprehensive analysis of inflammatory immune mediators in vitreoretinal diseases. *PLoS One*, 2009. 4(12): p. e8158.

[50] Itoi, K., et al., Relationship between diabetic macular edema and peripheral Th1/Th2 balance. *Ophthalmologica*, 2008. 222(4): p. 249-53.

[51] Chong, D. Y., et al., Interleukin-6 as a photoreceptor neuroprotectant in an experimental model of retinal detachment. *Invest. Ophthalmol. Vis. Sci.*, 2008. 49(7): p. 3193-200.

[52] Rothova, A., Inflammatory cystoid macular edema. *Curr. Opin. Ophthalmol.*, 2007. 18(6): p. 487-92.

[53] Rangasamy, S., P. G. McGuire, and A. Das, Diabetic retinopathy and inflammation: novel therapeutic targets. *Middle East Afr. J. Ophthalmol.*, 2012. 19(1): p. 52-9.

[54] Koss, M. J., et al., Comparison of cytokine levels from undiluted vitreous of untreated patients with retinal vein occlusion. *Acta Ophthalmol.*, 2012. 90(2): p. e98-e103.

[55] Kaneda, S., et al., Multivariate analyses of inflammatory cytokines in eyes with branch retinal vein occlusion: relationships to bevacizumab treatment. *Invest. Ophthalmol. Vis. Sci.*, 2011. 52(6): p. 2982-8.

[56] Roh, M. I., et al., Concentration of cytokines in the aqueous humor of patients with naive, recurrent and regressed CNV associated with amd after bevacizumab treatment. *Retina*, 2009. 29(4): p. 523-9.

[57] Liu, B., et al., Complement component C5a promotes expression of IL-22 and IL-17 from human T cells and its implication in age-related macular degeneration. *J. Transl. Med.*, 2011. 9: p. 1-12.
[58] Kuno, N. and S. Fujii, Biodegradable intraocular therapies for retinal disorders: progress to date. *Drugs Aging*, 2010. 27(2): p. 117-34.
[59] Graham, R. O. and G. A. Peyman, Intravitreal injection of dexamethasone. Treatment of experimentally induced endophthalmitis. *Arch. Ophthalmol.*, 1974. 92(2): p. 149-54.
[60] Irvine, W. D., et al., Endophthalmitis caused by gram-negative organisms. *Arch. Ophthalmol.*, 1992. 110(10): p. 1450-4.
[61] Park, S. S., et al., Effect of intravitreal dexamethasone in treatment of pneumococcal endophthalmitis in rabbits. *Arch. Ophthalmol.*, 1995. 113(10): p. 1324-9.
[62] Das, T., et al., Intravitreal dexamethasone in exogenous bacterial endophthalmitis: results of a prospective randomised study. *Br. J. Ophthalmol.*, 1999. 83(9): p. 1050-5.
[63] Gan, I. M., et al., Intravitreal dexamethasone as adjuvant in the treatment of postoperative endophthalmitis: a prospective randomized trial. *Graefes Arch. Clin. Exp. Ophthalmol.*, 2005. 243(12): p. 1200-5.
[64] Jacobs, D. J., et al., Intravitreal dexamethasone in the management of delayed-onset bleb-associated endophthalmitis. *Int. J. Inflam.*, 2012. 2012: p. 503912.
[65] Hall, E. F., et al., Adjunctive intravitreal dexamethasone in the treatment of acute endophthalmitis following cataract surgery. *Clin. Ophthalmol.*, 2008. 2(1): p. 139-45.
[66] Shah, G. K., et al., Visual outcomes following the use of intravitreal steroids in the treatment of postoperative endophthalmitis. *Ophthalmology*, 2000. 107(3): p. 486-9.
[67] Pollack, J. S. *ASRS pat survey*. 2004 [cited 2013 April 23]; Available from: http://www.asrs.org/.
[68] Ryan, S. J., et al., *Retina*. 4th ed. 2012.
[69] Tano, Y., et al., Inhibition of intraocular proliferations with intravitreal corticosteroids. *Am. J. Ophthalmol.*, 1980. 89(1): p. 131-6.
[70] Blankenship, G. W., Evaluation of a single intravitreal injection of dexamethasone phosphate in vitrectomy surgery for diabetic retinopathy complications. *Graefes Arch. Clin. Exp. Ophthalmol.*, 1991. 229(1): p. 62-5.

[71] Chalam, K. V., S. Malkani, and V. A. Shah, Intravitreal dexamethasone effectively reduces postoperative inflammation after vitreoretinal surgery. *Ophthalmic Surg. Lasers Imaging*, 2003. 34(3): p. 188-92.

[72] Bakri, S. J., et al., Same-day triple therapy with photodynamic therapy, intravitreal dexamethasone, and bevacizumab in wet age-related macular degeneration. *Retina*, 2009. 29(5): p. 573-8.

[73] Augustin, A., Triple therapy for age-related macular degeneration. *Retina*, 2009. 29(6 Suppl): p. S8-11.

[74] Yip, P. P., et al., Triple therapy for neovascular age-related macular degeneration using single-session photodynamic therapy combined with intravitreal bevacizumab and triamcinolone. *Br. J. Ophthalmol.*, 2009. 93(6): p. 754-8.

[75] Forte, R., et al., Intravitreal ranibizumab and bevacizumab in combination with full-fluence verteporfin therapy and dexamethasone for exudative age-related macular degeneration. *Ophthalmic Res.*, 2011. 45(3): p. 129-34.

[76] Koss, M. J., et al., Quadruple therapy leads to a sustained improvement of vision in patients with wet age-related macular degeneration. *Ophthalmologica*, 2011. 226(2): p. 45-50.

[77] Boyer, D. S., et al., Dexamethasone intravitreal implant for treatment of diabetic macular edema in vitrectomized patients. *Retina*, 2011. 31(5): p. 915-23.

[78] Ingerman, A. M., MSC and D. Dewey-Mattia (2010) Emerging Treatments for Diabetic Macular Edema: A review of agents in clinical trials. *Retina Today*.

[79] Kuppermann, B. D., et al., Randomized controlled study of an intravitreous dexamethasone drug delivery system in patients with persistent macular edema. *Arch. Ophthalmol.*, 2007. 125(3): p. 309-17.

[80] Haller, J. A., et al., Randomized controlled trial of an intravitreous dexamethasone drug delivery system in patients with diabetic macular edema. *Arch. Ophthalmol.*, 2010. 128(3): p. 289-96.

[81] Querques, L., et al., Repeated intravitreal dexamethasone implant (Ozurdex(R)) for retinal vein occlusion. *Ophthalmologica*, 2013. 229(1): p. 21-5.

[82] Moisseiev, E., et al., Long-term evaluation of patients treated with dexamethasone intravitreal implant for macular edema due to retinal vein occlusion. *Eye* (Lond), 2013. 27(1): p. 65-71.

[83] Matonti, F., et al., Repeated treatment for macular edema in vein occlusion by intravitreal implant of dexamethasone. *Case Rep. Ophthalmol.*, 2012. 3(3): p. 339-42.

[84] Lobo, C., Pseudophakic cystoid macular edema. *Ophthalmologica*, 2012. 227(2): p. 61-7.

[85] Comyn, O., S. L. Lightman, and P. G. Hykin, Corticosteroid intravitreal implants vs. ranibizumab for the treatment of vitreoretinal disease. *Curr. Opin. Ophthalmol.*, 2013. 24(3): p. 248-54.

[86] Yonekawa, Y. and I. K. Kim, Pseudophakic cystoid macular edema. *Curr. Opin. Ophthalmol.*, 2012. 23(1): p. 26-32.

[87] Albert, D. M., *Principles and Practice of Ophthalmology*, D. M. Albert and F. A. Jakobiec, Editors. 2000, W. B. Saunders Company: Philadelphia, PA.

[88] Lowder, C., et al., Dexamethasone intravitreal implant for noninfectious intermediate or posterior uveitis. *Arch. Ophthalmol.*, 2011. 129(5): p. 545-53.

[89] Arcinue, C. A., O. M. Ceron, and C. S. Foster, A Comparison Between the Fluocinolone Acetonide (Retisert) and Dexamethasone (Ozurdex) Intravitreal Implants in Uveitis. *J. Ocul. Pharmacol. Ther.*, 2013.

[90] Kishore, K., M. D. Conway, and G. A. Peyman, Intravitreal clindamycin and dexamethasone for toxoplasmic retinochoroiditis. *Ophthalmic Surg. Lasers*, 2001. 32(3): p. 183-92.

[91] Lasave, A. F., et al., Intravitreal clindamycin and dexamethasone for zone 1 toxoplasmic retinochoroiditis at twenty-four months. *Ophthalmology*, 2010. 117(9): p. 1831-8.

[92] Yeh, S. and R. B. Nussenblatt, Fluocinolone acetonide for the treatment of uveitis: weighing the balance between local and systemic immunosuppression. *Arch. Ophthalmol.*, 2008. 126(9): p. 1287-9.

[93] Haller, J. A., et al., Randomized, sham-controlled trial of dexamethasone intravitreal implant in patients with macular edema due to retinal vein occlusion. *Ophthalmology*, 2010. 117(6): p. 1134-1146 e3.

[94] Haller, J. A., et al., Dexamethasone intravitreal implant in patients with macular edema related to branch or central retinal vein occlusion twelve-month study results. *Ophthalmology*, 2011. 118(12): p. 2453-60.

[95] Kishore, S. A. and S. Schaal, Management of anterior chamber dislocation of dexamethasone implant. *Ocul. Immunol. Inflamm.*, 2013. 21(1): p. 70-1.

[96] Malcles, A., et al., [Anterior chamber migration of intravitreal dexamethasone implant (Ozurdex((R))) in pseudophakic eyes: Report of three cases.]. *J. Fr. Ophtalmol.*, 2013.

[97] Endophthalmitis Vitrectomy Study Group, Results of the endophthalmitis vitrectomy study. A randomized trial of immediate vitrectomy and of intravenous antibiotics for the treatment of postoperative bacterial endophthalmitis. Arch Ophthalmol, 1995. 113:p.479–496.

In: Dexamethasone
Editors: A. Sauvage and M. Levy
ISBN: 978-1-62808-405-4

Chapter IV

Anti-Tumor Activities of Dexamethasone

***Hitoshi Ishiguro*[1,2], *Takashi Kawahara*[1,2], *Yi Li*[1,3] *and Hiroshi Miyamoto*[1,2,*]**

[1]Department of Pathology and Laboratory Medicine, University of Rochester Medical Center, New York, US

[2]Departments of Pathology and Urology, Johns Hopkins University School of Medicine, Maryland, US

[3]Department of Urology, 2nd Affiliated Hospital, Zhejiang University School of Medicine, Hangzhou, China

Abstract

It is well known that dexamethasone (DEX) and other glucocorticoids are of great value in the treatment of various pathologic conditions, including inflammatory disorders and autoimmune diseases. In patients with solid tumors, a glucocorticoid is often prescribed, for instance, to reduce side effects of chemotherapeutic agents and to improve cachectic conditions. DEX, given alone or in combination with other drugs, has also been clinically used as a direct chemotherapeutic agent, primarily in hematological malignancies such as multiple myeloma

* E-mail: hmiyamo1@jhmi.edu.

and acute lymphocytic leukemia. In contrast, cytotoxic activities of DEX on solid tumors remain poorly characterized. Nonetheless, recent experimental data have suggested its direct effects on cell growth of solid tumors, such as prostate and bladder carcinomas. Indeed, in patients with castration-resistant prostate cancer, DEX treatment with or without docetaxel has been shown to prolong their survival. This chapter reviews clinical and molecular evidence supporting anti-tumor properties of DEX.

Introduction

Chemotherapy and radiotherapy for cancer often have severe side effects that may limit their efficacy. Due to their ability to reduce acute toxicity, particularly hyperemesis during systemic chemotherapy, as well as to protect normal tissue against the long-term effects of genotoxic drugs, glucocorticoids (GCs), such as dexamethasone (DEX), prednisone/prednisolone, and hydrocortisone, are frequently used in cancer patients [1]. GCs are also known to improve cachectic conditions (*e.g.* fatigue, poor appetite, weight loss, pain) in patients with end-stage disease. Thus, GCs are often given to patients with solid tumor without expecting their anti-tumor activities. GC is indeed involved in almost every cellular, molecular, and physiologic network of the organism and represents one of the most commonly prescribed drugs often employed in the treatment of inflammatory and autoimmune disorders.

Meanwhile, several GCs, including DEX, have been clinically used as cytotoxic agents, predominantly for lymphomas. GCs have also been applied to the treatment of castration-resistant prostate cancer (CRPC), whereas cytotoxic activities of DEX on other types of solid tumors remain poorly characterized. However, there is an increasing amount of experimental evidence suggesting the direct effects of DEX on cell growth of solid tumors.

In general, GC-bound glucocorticoid receptor (GR) in susceptible cells forms complexes, translocates into the nucleus, and binds to GC response elements, resulting in induction of gene transcription [2]. The activated GC-GR complex also interacts with transcription factors, such as nuclear factor (NF)-κB and activator protein 1 (AP-1), and other genes, such as *c-myc* proto-oncogene, most of which are involved in cell proliferation/survival and cell cycle regulation [3]. These mechanisms ultimately, for instance, promote apoptosis. This chapter aims to provide an overview of not only clinical studies showing the benefit of DEX for the treatment of malignancies but also molecular data supporting anti-tumor properties of DEX.

Clinical Evidence of Anti-Tumor Effects

As described, DEX is known to reduce acute toxicity of cytotoxic drugs and has therefore been widely used as comedication in patients with solid tumor. Of note was that co-treatment with DEX could reduce the sensitivity of chemotherapeutic drugs, including cisplatin, paclitaxel, trastuzumab, and gemcitabine [4-7]. On the other hand, DEX showing potent proapoptotic properties predominantly in lymphoma cells [8] has also been clinically used as a cytotoxic agent. Indeed, GCs have been being used in the treatment of childhood leukemia for several decades, and they have become one of the most common drugs included in almost all chemotherapy protocols for lymphoid malignancies.

In this section, we describe the clinical data indicating anti-tumor effects of DEX primarily on hematological malignancies and prostate cancer.

Multiple Myeloma

Multiple myeloma is a malignant neoplasm of plasma cells that accumulate in bone marrow, leading to bone destruction and marrow failure. It is estimated that 22,350 new cases of multiple myeloma will be diagnosed in the United States in 2013 and that 10,710 deaths from this disease will occur [9].

Multiple myeloma is the most notable disease using DEX for anti-tumor activity. Since 1960s, melphalan-prednisone (MP) has been used for multiple myeloma and remains a widely accepted treatment option [10,11]. After 1990s, DEX is also frequently used for multiple myeloma, both in untreated patients and at relapse [11,12]. The common chemotherapy regimens include MP, vincristine-doxorubicin-DEX (VAD), vincristine-mitoxantrone-DEX (VND), and their combinations (*e.g.* MP/VAD, MP/VND) [11-13]. The use of high-dose chemotherapy followed by autologous stem cell transplantation (ASCT) has improved patient outcomes and is now considered the standard of care for symptomatic multiple myeloma patients younger than 65 years [14,15]. Recently, thalidomide combined with DEX followed by ASCT has successfully been introduced in the new target therapy of multiple myeloma with high efficacy [15]. Furthermore, induction with thalidomide plus DEX did not compromise the viability of stem cell collection for subsequent ASCT.

Monotherapy with high-dose DEX shows anti-tumor effects on the progression of multiple myeloma and has also been used for select elderly patients with, for instance, renal failure [10,15]. However, due to lower response rate of monotherapy compared to the combination therapy, DEX is commonly used in combination with other chemotherapeutic drugs.

Acute Lymphoblastic Leukemia (ALL)

ALL is the most common childhood cancer and more than 80% of children with ALL can be cured by current systemic chemotherapy [16]. GCs have been included in almost all treatment regimens for childhood ALL for several decades; initially cortisone and adrenocorticotropic hormone were used, later prednisone, and occasionally DEX [17]. GCs further suppress the proliferation of various types of cells, including ALL, via regulation of cell cycle [8,18]. GC sensitivity *in vivo* as well as *in vitro* is known as a major prognostic factor in childhood ALL [8,19].

Emerging evidence supports that DEX has marked cytotoxic activity, with response rates higher than any other single drug [17]. However, despite the effectiveness of GCs in ALL, these drugs are not curative when used as a single agent. In addition, a strong cross-resistance to DEX and prednisone, although DEX is much more active than prednisone, has been observed in ALL cells [20].

Prostate Cancer

Prostate cancer is the most commonly diagnosed malignancy in men in the United States [9] and is one of solid tumors in which DEX has clinically shown an anti-tumor effect.

Although most of patients even with metastatic prostate cancer respond to initial androgen deprivation therapy, they ultimately develop progressive disease with androgen-independent tumor [21]. Most of prostate cancer tissues have indeed been found to show low or absent GR expression [22], whereas the levels of GR protein are augmented following androgen deprivation therapy [23].

Previous chemotherapy trials in CRPC resulted in low response rates and minimal survival impact, but introduction of docetaxel improved the outcome of chemotherapy in CRPC patients [24]. DEX has been clinically used not only as a single anti-tumor agent but also in combination with other chemotherapeutic drugs in prostate cancer

It is likely that there are two roles of anti-tumor effects of DEX in the treatment of CRPC: systemic and focal functions. These include: 1) suppression of androgens derived from the adrenal; 2) anti-inflammatory effects [*e.g.* inhibition of interleukin (IL)-6 and cyclooxygenase-2]; and 3) anti-stress effects (*e.g.* induction of cyclin-dependent kinase inhibitors, p21 and p27).

Table 1. Glucocorticoid monotherapy in CRPC

Year [Ref]	N	Daily Dose	PSA Response (decline >50%)	Remarks
Prednisone				
1989 [26]	37	7.5-10 mg	NA	38% improvement in pain
1996 [30]	81	5 mg	22%	12.3% symptomatic improvement
1998 [32]	29	10 mg	34%	
2000 [35]	60	5 mg	24%	
2001 [38]	101	5 mg	21%	50% subjective response
2006 [40]	15	10 mg	27%	
Hydrocortisone				
1995 [29]	30	40 mg	20%	
1999 [33]	123	40 mg	22%	
2000 [36]	231	40 mg	16%	28% improvement in pain
Dexamethasone				
1990 [27]	29	0.75 mg	NA	2 cases with objective response
1995 [28]	38	0.75 mg	61%	63% symptomatic improvement
1998 [31]	7	0.5-1.5 mg	57%	All responders were PSA decline >90%
2000 [34]	37	0.5-2.0 mg	62%	61% improvement in pain
2001 [37]	19	1.5 mg	28%	
2002 [39]	27	1.5 mg	59%	
2008 [41]	99	0.5-1.5 mg	40%	

The clinical efficacy of GC monotherapy for CRPC has been reported since 1950s [25-41]. Various GCs, including prednisone, hydrocortisone, and DEX, as minimally toxic, low-cost therapy were assessed, showing considerable decreases in prostate-specific antigen (PSA) levels and apparent beneficial effects on subjective symptoms in patients with CRPC (Table 1). In these studies, rates of PSA response (*i.e.* decline of greater than 50%) to DEX (28-62%) were shown to be much higher than those to prednisone (21-34%) or hydrocortisone (16-22%). The dosage of DEX was ranged from 0.5 to 2.0 mg/day and severe toxicities of low-dose DEX were infrequently observed in these patients.

Docetaxel, currently the most widely used chemotherapeutic agent against CRPC, inhibits tumor growth via microtubule stabilization and bcl-2 inactivation, which leads to induction of apoptosis [42-44]. Prednisone has often been combined with docetaxel for the treatment of CRPC [44-46]. Instead, two recent reports showed that treatment with docetaxel and DEX resulted in a PSA decline of 50% or greater in 58% (42/72; with estramustine phosphate [47]) and 75% (6/8; with continuous luteinizing hormone-releasing hormone analog [48]) of patients with CRPC. In addition, pretreatment of DEX prior to docetaxel administration likely reduced the incidence of hypersensitivity reactions and fluid retention associated with docetaxel [49]. The most common toxicity of docetaxel plus DEX includes neutropenia (mostly grades 1-2) [47,48].

Experimental Evidence of Anti-Tumor Effects in Solid Tumors

Recent *in vitro* and *in vivo* studies have suggested a pivotal role of DEX treatment in the suppression of tumor progression through the GR pathway in various types of solid tumor cells. However, DEX has been reported to regulate cell growth in a manner specific for cell/tissue types. Thus, in certain cell lines DEX did not affect or even did promote their growth. Furthermore, there are some controversies regarding the effects of DEX even in the same types of cells, and it is still necessary to clarify the mechanisms of tumor regression (or progression) by GR signals.

In this section, we focus on suppressive function of DEX on the progression of solid tumors. Table 2 summarizes reported inhibitory effects of DEX on the growth of different types of cancer cell lines.

Table 2. Inhibitory effects of DEX in various types of cancer cells

Cancer Type	Related Molecules	Function	Reference
Urinary Bladder	MMP-2 ↓	Invasion ↓	[52]
	MMP-9 ↓	Invasion ↓	[52]
	IL-6 ↓	Invasion ↓	[52]
	VEGF ↓	Invasion ↓	[52]
	IκBα ↑	Invasion ↓	[52]
	NF-κB (nuclear) ↓	Invasion ↓	[52]
Brain	angiopoietin 2 ↓	Proliferation ↓	[54]
	MMP-2 ↓	Proliferation ↓ Invasion ↓	[54,56]
Breast	SULT1E1 ↑	deactivation of estrogens	[58]
	ABCG2 ↓	chemotherapy effect ↑	[59]
Lung	cyclin D1 ↓	Proliferation ↓	[61]
	p21 ↑	Proliferation ↓	[61]
	c-myc ↓	Proliferation ↓	[61]
	BAD ↑	Proliferation ↓	[62]
	BAX ↑	Proliferation ↓	[62]
	cyclin D2 ↓	Proliferation ↓	[62]
Prostate	IL-6 ↓	Proliferation ↓	[64]
	IL-8 ↓	Angiogenesis ↓	[67,69]
	NF-κB ↓	Angiogenesis ↓	[69]
	IκBα ↑	Proliferation ↓	[64]
	CXCL1 ↓	Angiogenesis ↓	[69]
	VEGF ↓	Angiogenesis ↓	[67]
	VEGF-C ↓	lymphangiogenesis ↓	[68]
	ERK1/2	Proliferation ↓	[66]
	cyclin D1 ↓	Proliferation ↓	[66]
Cervix	p57 ↑	Proliferation ↓	[71]
	NF-κB ↓	chemotherapy effect ↑	[72]
Oral Cavity, Head, and Neck	uPA ↓	Invasion ↓	[73]
	PAI-1 ↑	Invasion ↓	[73]
	VEGF ↓	Angiogenesis ↓	[75]
Stomach	α1/β1 integrin ↑	cell adhesion ↑	[76]
Kidney	IL-6 ↓	Proliferation ↓	[78]
	IL-8 ↓	Angiogenesis ↓	[78]
	NF-κB ↓	Proliferation ↓	[78]
	VEGF ↓	Angiogenesis ↓	[77,78]
Pancreas	IL-8 ↓	Invasion ↓	[79]
	NF-κB ↓	Invasion ↓	[79]

Urinary Bladder Cancer

Prolonged systemic use of GC is known to correlate with increased risk of bladder cancer [50], although detailed functions of GCs in bladder tumorigenesis remain unclear. DEX-mediated promotion of cell proliferation and inhibition of anti-proliferative effects of chemotherapeutic agents via prevention of apoptosis have also been reported in bladder cancer [51,52]. In contrast, we recently demonstrated that DEX strongly suppressed bladder cancer cell invasion and metastasis *in vitro* and *in vivo* [52]. DEX treatment also resulted in down-regulation of invasion/metastasis-related molecules, including matrix metalloproteinase (MMP)-2, MMP-9, vascular endothelial growth factor (VEGF), and IL-6. We additionally showed an increase in IκBα level and a blockade of nuclear translocation of NF-κB by DEX as well as DEX-induced mesenchymal-to-epithelial transition, all of which may be central mechanisms involved in GR-mediated inhibition of bladder tumor progression. In these cell line models, DEX effects were abolished by a GR antagonist or GR knock-down via RNA interference. Furthermore, our immunohistochemical study in radical cystectomy specimens revealed lower expression of GR in tumor than in benign urothelium and a tendency to associate strong GR expression with better prognosis [52]. Thus, it is likely that DEX-activated GR signals promote bladder cancer cell proliferation yet repress cell invasion and metastasis. More recently, we found that several other GCs exhibited strong inhibition of cell invasion similar to that of DEX while they had no significant stimulatory effects on cell viability (Ishiguro et al., unpublished data).

Brain Tumor

Patients with brain tumor are often treated with DEX primarily to ameliorate cerebral edema. Nonetheless, Kaup et al. first showed the findings suggestive of a direct effect of DEX on the proliferation of three glioblastoma lines [53]. The response to different doses/times of DEX treatment appeared to be cell line-specific. Villeneuve et al. then showed that DEX treatment reduced the growth of orthotopically implanted glioblastoma cells in mice but did not significantly inhibit the viability of the cells *in vitro* [54]. DEX treatment also resulted in reduction of vascular enlargement, presumably via down-regulation of angiogenic factors. In addition, using mouse xenograft models with another glioma cell line (U87MG) as well as other types of cancer lines (breast, colon, lung), Wang et al. demonstrated that DEX pretreatment enhanced the anti-tumor activity of chemotherapeutic agents and increased their accumulation in tumors while DEX alone showed minimal anti-tumor effects [55]. On the other hand, DEX was shown to decrease MMP-2 secretion and invasiveness in U87MG cells through mitogen activated protein kinase phosphatase-1 induction [56].

Breast Cancer

Breast cancer, like prostate cancer, is an endocrine-related neoplasm, and estrogens promote its progression. In an estrogen receptor-positive breast cancer line, DEX antagonized estrogens resulting in inhibition of estrogen-induced cell growth [57]. Gong et al. further revealed the metabolism-based mechanism of anti-estrogenic activity of DEX [58]. DEX induced the expression and activity of estrogen sulfotransferase (SULT1E1), leading to metabolic deactivation of estrogens, and could lower circulating estrogens. In two breast cancer cell lines, DEX was also shown to increase the sensitivity to chemotherapeutic drugs [55,59], possibly via down-regulation of the breast cancer resistance protein ABCG2, a member of ATP-binding cassette family, in cancer cells [59].

Lung Cancer

GR was found to express roughly half of non-small cell lung cancer tissues, and patients with GR-positive tumor had significantly more favorable outcomes than those with GR-negative tumor [60]. The same study also showed that DEX regulated the growth of lung cancer cells and the sensitivity to different anti-cancer drugs *in vitro* [60]. Interestingly, the effects of DEX on cell proliferation (stimulation *vs.* inhibition) and chemosensitivity (increase *vs.* decrease) were cell line-specific. Furthermore, other studies demonstrated suppressive effects of DEX on cell proliferation of non-small cell lung cancer via inhibition of the extracellular signal-related kinase (ERK) pathway and cell cycle regulators [61] as well as on that of small cell lung cancer via up-regulation of proapoptotic genes [62].

Prostate Cancer

As described above, DEX, with or without other cytotoxic agents, has been clinically used especially for the treatment of CRPC. In addition to its direct effect in cancer cells, DEX is known to reduce adrenal androgen production [63]. Nishimura et al. first demonstrated molecular evidence indicating a mechanism for anti-tumor effects of DEX in prostate cancer [64]. DEX treatment inhibited CRPC cell growth through the disruption of the NF-κB/IL-6 pathway (*i.e.* increasing IκBα levels and cytosolic accumulation of NF-κB, decreasing IL-6 secretion). Indeed, DEX therapy markedly decreased serum levels of IL-6 in patients with CRPC who responded to DEX, but not in non-responders [65]. DEX was also shown to inhibit an androgen receptor-negative prostate cancer cell proliferation at the G0/G1 phase by down-regulating ERK1/2 and cyclin D1 [66]. Other mechanisms of suppressive effects of DEX on CRPC growth included inhibitions of tumor angiogenesis by down-regulating VEGF and IL-8 [67] and lymphangiogenesis by down-regulating VEGF-C [68], all of which were mediated through the GR pathway. Moreover, DEX attenuated docetaxel-induced NF-κB and AP-1 activation in prostate cancer cells and thus potentiated the anti-angiogenic activity of docetaxel [69].

Other Malignancies

Anti-tumor effects of DEX have been indicated in other types of solid malignancies.

In cervical cancer lines, DEX inhibited cell proliferation [70] via transcriptional induction of p57 [71] and enhanced the cytotoxic activity of cisplatin by inhibiting NF-κB activation [72].

In oral squamous cell carcinoma lines, DEX inhibited cell invasion via decreasing urokinase-type plasminogen activator (uPA) and increasing the uPA inhibitor plasminogen activator inhibitor-I (PAI-1) production [73], which might be further mediated by AP-1 [74]. In head and neck squamous cancer lines, DEX treatment also resulted in inhibition of cell proliferation and VEGF secretion mediated by signal transducer and activator of transcription 3 (STAT3) [75].

In a gastric cancer line, DEX inhibited epidermal growth factor-induced cell migration by enhancing cell adhesion to the extracellular matrix via α1 and β1 integrin subunits, possibly forming the α1β1 heterodimer [76].

In renal cell carcinoma cells, DEX inactivated NF-κB, reduced the expression and secretion of its downstream products, including VEGF, IL-6, and IL-8, and thereby inhibited their growth [77,78].

In pancreatic cancer lines, DEX did not show a significant anti-proliferative effect *in vitro* yet strongly suppressed invasiveness *in vitro* and tumor growth/metastasis in a mouse orthotopic xenograft model, associated with inhibition of NF-κB activity and IL-8 secretion [79].

In a rat hepatoma line, DEX inhibited cell viability by inducing apoptosis and NF-κB inactivation [80].

In a colon cancer line, as described earlier, pretreatment with DEX enhanced therapeutic effects of carboplatin and gemcitabine *in vivo* [55].

In melanoma, GR expression was found to be down-regulated, compared to normal skin or nevus, and high doses of DEX inhibited cell growth, but not cell migration, *in vitro* [81]. In osteosarcoma lines with exogenously overexpressing GR, DEX treatment resulted in inhibition of cell proliferation and G1 cell cycle arrest [82].

Conclusion

DEX is often prescribed during systemic chemotherapy for the purpose of reducing acute and late phase side effects of cytotoxic drugs. On the other hand, DEX possessing direct anti-tumor activities is clinically used in some hematological tumors and CRPC as monotherapy or in combination with other chemotherapeutic agents. Disadvantages of its clinical use include: 1) increasing subsequent risks of other malignancies; 2) decreasing the chemosensitivity to some drugs; and 3) inducing various side effects, such as a rise in blood glucose level, osteoporosis, and hypertension.

Recent experimental evidence also suggests that DEX suppresses the progression of solid tumors directly and indirectly in a manner specific for cell types. Thus, in a variety of malignancies DEX treatment is shown to result in a significantly reduced cell proliferation, invasion, and metastasis *in vitro* and *in vivo*. Further investigation is still required to clarify the detailed mechanisms of direct anti-tumor effects of DEX, which may in turn identify cancer patients who benefit from treatment with DEX.

References

[1] Basch E, Prestrud A. A, Hesketh P. J, Kris M. G, Feyer P. C, Somerfield M. R, et al. Antiemetics: American Society of Clinical Oncology clinical practice guideline update. *J. Clin. Oncol.* 29: 4189-4198, 2011.

[2] Grad I, Picard D. The glucocorticoid responses are shaped by molecular chaperones. *Mol. Cell. Endocrinol.* 275: 2-12, 2007. ("Cell." for "Cellular")

[3] De Bosscher K, Vanden Berghe W, Haegeman G. The interplay between the glucocorticoid receptor and nuclear factor-κB or activator protein-1: Molecular mechanisms for gene repression. *Endocr. Rev.* 24: 488-522, 2003.

[4] Sumikawa T, Shigeoka Y, Igishi T, Suyama H, Yamasaki A, Hashimoto K, et al. Dexamethasone interferes with trastuzumab-induced cell growth inhibition through restoration of AKT activity in BT-474 breast cancer cells. *Int. J. Oncol.* 32: 683-688, 2008.

[5] Qian Y-H, Xiao Q, Chen H, Xu J. Dexamethasone inhibits camptothecin-induced apoptosis in C6-glioma via activation of Stat5/Bcl-xL pathway. *Biochim. Biophys. Acta*. 1793: 764-771, 2009.

[6] Chen Y-X, Wang Y, Fu C-C, Diao F, Song L-N, Li Z-B, et al. Dexamethasone enhances cell resistance to chemotherapy by increasing adhesion to extracellular matrix in human ovarian cancer cells. *Endocr. Relat. Cancer.* 17: 39-50, 2010.

[7] Ge H, Ni S, Wang X, Xu N, Liu Y, Wang L, et al. Dexamethasone reduces sensitivity to cisplatin by blunting p53-dependent cellular senescence in non-small cell lung cancer. *PLoS One*. 7: e51821, 2012.

[8] Schmidt S, Rainer J, Ploner C, Presul E, Riml S, Kofler R. Glucocorticoid-induced apoptosis and glucocorticoid resistance: molecular mechanisms and clinical relevance. *Cell Death Differ.* 11 (Suppl 1): S45-S55, 2004.

[9] Siegel R, Naishadham D, Jemal A. Cancer statistics, 2013. *CA Cancer J. Clin.* 63: 11-30, 2013.

[10] Alexanian R, Haut A, Khan A. U, Lane M, McKelvey E. M, Migliore P. J, et al. Treatment for multiple myeloma. Combination chemotherapy with different melphalan dose regimens. *JAMA* 208: 1680-1685, 1969.

[11] Facon T, Mary J. Y, Pégourie B, Attal M, Renaud M, Sadoun A, et al. Dexamethasone-based regimens versus melphalan-prednisone for

elderly multiple myeloma patients ineligible for high-dose therapy. *Blood*. 107: 1292-1298, 2006.

[12] Alexanian R, Dimopoulos M. A, Delasalle K, Barlogie B. Primary dexamethasone treatment of multiple myeloma. *Blood*. 80: 887-890, 1992.

[13] Cavo M, Benni M, Ronconi S, Fiacchini M, Gozzetti A, Zamaqni E, et al. Melphalan-prednisone versus alternating combination VAD/MP or VND/MP as primary therapy for multiple myeloma: final analysis of a randomized clinical study. *Hematologica*. 87: 934-942, 2002.

[14] Attal M, Harousseau JL, Stoppa A. M, Sotto J. J, Fuzibet J. G, Rossi J. F, et al. A prospective, randomized trial of autologous bone marrow transplantation and chemotherapy in multiple myeloma. *N. Engl. J. Med.* 335: 91-97, 1996.

[15] Chen H-F, Li Z-Y, Tang J-Q, Shen H-S, Cui Q-Y, Ren Y-Y, et al. Clinical study of thalidomide combined with dexamethasone for the treatment of elderly patients with newly diagnosed multiple myeloma. *Asian Pac. J. Cancer Prev*. 13: 4777-4781, 2012.

[16] Mattano L. A Jr., Devidas M, Nachman J. B, Sather H. N, Hunger S. P, Steinherz P. G. Effect of alternate-week versus continuous dexamethasone scheduling on the risk of osteonecrosis in paediatric patients with acute lymphoblastic leukaemia: Results from the CCG-1961 randomised cohort trial. *Lancet Oncol*. 13: 906-915, 2012.

[17] Kaspers G. J, Pieters R, Klumper E, De Waal F. C, Veerman A. J. Glucocorticoid resistance in childhood leukemia. Leuk. *Lymphoma*. 13: 187-201, 1994.

[18] Renner K, Ausserlechner M. J, Kofler R. A conceptual view on glucocorticoid-lnduced apoptosis, cell cycle arrest and glucocorticoid resistance in lymphoblastic leukemia. *Curr. Mol. Med*. 3: 707-717, 2003.

[19] Tissing W. J, Meijerink J. P, den Boer M. L, Pieters R. Molecular determinants of glucocorticoid sensitivity and resistance in acute lymphoblastic leukemia. *Leukemia*. 17: 17-25, 2003.

[20] Bostrom B. C, Sensel M. R, Sather H. N, Gaynon P. S, La M. K, Johnston K, et al. Dexamethasone versus prednisone and daily oral versus weekly intravenous mercaptopurine for patients with standard-risk acute lymphoblastic leukemia: A report from Children's Cancer Group. *Blood*. 101: 3809-3817, 2003.

[21] Singer E. A, Golijanin D. J, Miyamoto H, Messing E. M. Androgen deprivation therapy for prostate cancer. *Expert Opin. Pharmacother*. 9: 211-228, 2008.

[22] Yemelyanov A, Czwornog J, Chebotaev D, Karseladze A, Kulevitch E, Yang X, et al. Tumor suppressor activity of glucocorticoid receptor in the prostate. *Oncogene.* 26: 1885-1896, 2007.

[23] Szmulewitz R. Z, Chung E, Al-Ahmadie H, Daniel S, Kocherginsky M, Razmaria A, et al. Serum/glucocorticoid-regulated kinase 1 expression in primary human prostate cancers. *Prostate.* 72: 157-164, 2012.

[24] Millikan R. E. Chemotherapy of advanced prostatic carcinoma. *Semin. Oncol.* 26: 185-191, 1999.

[25] Miller G. M, Hinman F Jr. Cortisone treatment in advanced carcinoma of the prostate. *J. Urol.* 72: 485-496, 1954.

[26] Tannock I, Gospodarowicz M, Meakin W, Panzarella T, Stewart L, Rider W. Treatment of metastatic prostatic cancer with low-dose prednisone: evaluation of pain and quality of life as pragmatic indices of response. *J. Clin. Oncol.* 7: 590-597, 1989.

[27] Patel S. R, Kvols L. K, Hahn R. G, Windschitl H, Levitt R, Therneau T. A phase II randomized trial of megestrol acetate or dexamethasone in the treatment of hormonally refractory advanced carcinoma of the prostate. *Cancer.* 66: 655-658, 1990.

[28] Storlie J. A, Buckner J. C, Wiseman G. A, Burch P. A, Hartmann L. C, Richardson R. L. Prostate specific antigen levels and clinical response to low dose dexamethasone for hormone-refractory metastatic prostate carcinoma. *Cancer.* 76: 96-100, 1995.

[29] Kelly W. K, Curley T, Leibretz C, Dnistrian A, Schwartz M, Scher H. I. Prospective evaluation of hydrocortisone and suramin in patients with androgen-independent prostate cancer. *J. Clin. Oncol.* 13: 2208-2213, 1995.

[30] Tannock I. F, Osoba D, Stockler M. R, Ernst D. S, Neville A. J, Moore M. J, et al. Chemotherapy with mitoxantrone plus prednisone or prednisone alone for symptomatic hormone-resistant prostate cancer: a Canadian randomized trial with palliative end points. *J. Clin. Oncol.* 14: 1756-1764, 1996.

[31] Nishiyama T, Terunuma M. Hormone/antihormone withdrawal and dexamethasone for hormone-refractory prostate cancer. *Int. J. Urol.* 5: 44-47, 1998.

[32] Sartor O, Weinberger M, Moore A, Li A, Figg W. D. Effect of prednisone on prostate-specific antigen in patients with hormone-refractory prostate cancer. *Urology.* 52: 252-256, 1998.

[33] Kantoff P. W, Halabi S, Conaway M, Picus J, Kirshner J, Hars V, et al. Hydrocortisone with or without mitoxantrone in men with hormone-

refractory prostate cancer: results of the cancer and leukemia group B 9182 study. *J. Clin. Oncol.* 17: 2506-2513, 1999.

[34] Nishimura K, Nonomura N, Yasunaga Y, Takaha N, Inoue H, Sugao H, et al. Low doses of oral dexamethasone for hormone-refractory prostate carcinoma. *Cancer.* 89: 2570-2576, 2000.

[35] Berry W, Dakhil S, Modiano M, Gregurich M, Asmar L. Phase III study of mitoxantrone plus low dose prednisone versus low dose prednisone alone in patients with asymptomatic hormone refractory prostate cancer. *J. Urol.* 168: 2439-2443, 2002.

[36] Small E. J, Meyer M, Marshall M. E, Reyno L. M, Meyers F. J, Natale R. B, et al. Suramin therapy for patients with symptomatic hormone-refractory prostate cancer: results of a randomized phase III trial comparing suramin plus hydrocortisone to placebo plus hydrocortisone. *J. Clin. Oncol.* 18: 1440-1450, 2000.

[37] Saika T, Kusaka N, Tsushima T, Yamato T, Ohashi T, Suyama B, et al. Treatment of androgen-independent prostate cancer with dexamethasone: a prospective study in stage D2 patients. *Int. J. Urol.* 8: 290-294, 2001.

[38] Fossa S. D, Slee P. H, Brausi M, Horenblas S, Hall R. R, Hetherington J. W, et al. Flutamide versus prednisone in patients with prostate cancer symptomatically progressing after androgen-ablative therapy: a phase III study of the European organization for research and treatment of cancer genitourinary group. *J. Clin. Oncol.* 19: 62-71, 2001.

[39] Morioka M, Kobayashi T, Furukawa Y, Jo Y, Shinkai M, Matsuki T, et al. Prostate-specific antigen levels and prognosis in patients with hormone-refractory prostate cancer treated with low-dose dexamethasone. *Urol. Int.* 68: 10-15, 2002.

[40] Fuse H, Nozaki T, Fujiuchi Y, Mizuno I, Nagakawa O, Okumura A. Treatment with prednisolone of hormone-refractory prostate cancer. *Arch. Androl.* 52: 35-38, 2006.

[41] Komiya A, Shimbo M, Suzuki H, Imamoto T, Kato T, Fukasawa S, et al. Oral low-dose dexamethasone for androgen-independent prostate cancer patients. *Oncol. Lett.* 1: 73-79, 2010.

[42] Diaz J. F, Andreu J. M. Assembly of purified GDP-tubulin into microtubules induced by taxol and taxotere: reversibility, ligand stoichiometry, and competition. *Biochemistry.* 32: 2747-2755, 1993.

[43] Haldar S, Basu A, Croce C. M. Bcl2 is the guardian of microtubule integrity. *Cancer Res.* 57: 229-233, 1997.

[44] Kawahara T, Miyoshi Y, Sekiguchi Z, Sano F, Hayashi N, Teranishi J, et al. Risk factors for metastatic castration-resistant prostate cancer (CRPC) predict long-term treatment with docetaxel. *PLoS One*. 7: e48186, 2012.

[45] Tannock I. F, de Wit R, Berry W. R, Horti J, Pluzanska A, Chi K. N, et al. Docetaxel plus prednisone or mitoxantrone plus prednisone for advanced prostate cancer. *N. Engl. J. Med*. 351: 1502-1512, 2004.

[46] Pond G. R, Armstrong A. J, Wood B. A, Brookes M, Leopold L, Berry W. R, et al. Evaluating the value of number of cycles of docetaxel and prednisone in men with metastatic castration-resistant prostate cancer. *Eur. Urol*. 61: 363-369, 2012.

[47] Hatano K, Nishimura K, Nakai Y, Yoshida T, Sato M, Kawashima A, et al. Weekly low-dose docetaxel combined with estramustine and dexamethasone for Japanese patients with metastatic casstration-resistant prostate cancer. *Int. J. Clin. Oncol*., 2012 (in press).

[48] Miyoshi Y, Uemura H, Nakamura M, Hasumi H, Sugiura S, Makiyama K, et al. Treatment of androgen-independent, hormone-refractory prostate cancer with docetaxel in Japanese patients. *Int. J. Clin. Oncol.* 10: 182-186, 2005.

[49] Weitzman A. L, Shelton G, Zuech N, Owen C. E, Judge T, Benson M, et al. Dexamethasone does not significantly contribute to the response rate of docetaxel and estramustine in androgen independent prostate cancer. *J. Urol*. 163: 834-837, 2000.

[50] Dietrich K, Schned A, Fertuny J, Heaney J, Marsit C, Kelsey K. T, et al. Glucocorticoid therapy and risk of bladder cancer. *Br. J. Cancer*. 101: 1316-1320, 2009.

[51] Zhang C, Mattern J, Haferkamp A, Pfitzenmaier J, Hohenfellner M, Rittgen W, et al. Corticosteroid-induced chemotherapy resistance in urological cancers. *Cancer Biol. Ther*. 5: 59-64, 2006.

[52] Zheng Y, Izumi K, Li Y, Ishiguro H, Miyamoto H. Contrary regulation of bladder cancer cell proliferation and invasion by dexamethasone-mediated glucocorticoid receptor signals. *Mol. Cancer Ther*. 11: 2621-2632, 2012.

[53] Kaup B, Schindler I, Knüpfer H, Schlenzka A, Preiss R, Knüpfer M. M. Time-dependent inhibition of glioblastoma cell proliferation by dexamethasone. *J. Neurooncol*. 51: 105-110, 2001.

[54] Villeneuve J, Galarneau H, Beaudet M. J, Tremblay P, Chernomoretz A, Vallières L. Reduced glioma growth following dexamethasone or anti-angiopoietin 2 treatment. *Brain Pathol.* 18: 401-414, 2008.

[55] Wang H, Li M, Rinehart J. J, Zhang R. Pretreatment with dexamethasone increases antitumor activity of carboplatin and gemcitabine in mice bearing human cancer xenografts: *in vivo* activity, pharmacokinetics, and clinical implications for cancer chemotherapy. *Clin. Cancer Res.* 10: 1633-1644, 2004.

[56] Lin Y-M, Jan H-J, Lee C-C, Tao H-Y, Shih Y-L, Wei H-W, et al. Dexamethasone reduced invasiveness of human malignant glioblastoma cells through a MAPK phosphatase-1 (MKP-1) dependent mechanism. *Eur. J. Pharmacol.* 593: 1-9, 2008.

[57] Zhou F, Bouillard B, Pharaboz-Joly M. O, Andre J. Nonclassical antiestrogenic actions of dexamethasone in variant MCF-7 human breast cancer cells in culture. *Mol. Cell. Endocrinol.* 66: 189-197, 1989.

[58] Gong H, Jarzynka M. J, Cole T. J, Lee J. H, Wada T, Zhang B, et al. Glucocorticoids antagonize estrogens by glucocorticoid receptor-mediated activation of estrogen sulfotransferase. *Cancer Res.* 68: 7386-7393, 2008.

[59] Honorat M, Mesnier A, Di Pietro A, Lin V, Cohen P, Dumontet C, et al. Dexamethasone down-regulates ABCG2 expression levels in breast cancer cells. *Biochem. Biophys. Res. Commun.* 375: 308-314, 2008.

[60] Lu Y-S, Lien H-C, Yeh P-Y, Kuo S-H, Chang W-C, Kuo M-L, et al. Glucocorticoid receptor expression in advanced non-small cell lung cancer: clinicopathological correlation and *in vitro* effect of glucocorticoid on cell growth and chemosensitivity. *Lung Cancer.* 53: 303-310, 2006.

[61] Greenberg A. K, Hu J, Basu S, Hay J, Reibman J, Yie TA, et al. Glucocorticoids inhibit lung cancer cell growth through both the extracellular signal-related kinase pathway and cell cycle regulators. *Am. J. Respir. Cell Mol. Biol.* 27: 320-328, 2002.

[62] Sommer P, Le Rouzic P, Gillingham H, Berry A, Kayahara M, Huynh T, et al. Glucocorticoid receptor overexpression exerts an antisurvival effect on human small cell lung cancer cells. *Oncogene. 26:* 7111-7121, 2007.

[63] Feldman B. J, Feldman D. The development of androgen-independent prostate cancer. *Nat. Rev. Cancer.* 1: 34-45, 2001.

[64] Nishimura K, Nonomura N, Satoh E, Harada Y, Nakayama M, Tokizane T, et al. Potential mechanism for the effects of dexamethasone on growth of androgen-independent prostate cancer. *J. Natl. Cancer Inst.* 93: 1739-1746, 2001.

[65] Akakura K, Suzuki H, Ueda T, Komiya A, Ichikawa T, Igarashi T, et al. Possible mechanism of dexamethasone therapy for prostate cancer: suppression of circulating level of interleukin-6. *Prostate.* 56: 106-109, 2003.
[66] Gao Q-Z, Lu J-J, Liu Z-D, Zhang H, Wang S-M, Xu H. Dexamethasone suppresses DU145 cell proliferation and cell cycle through inhibition of the extracellular signal-related kinase 1/2 pathway and cyclin D1 expression. *Asian J. Androl.* 10: 635-641, 2008.
[67] Yano A, Fujii Y, Iwai A, Kageyama Y, Kihara K. Glucocorticoids suppress tumor angiogenesis and *in vivo* growth of prostate cancer cells. *Clin. Cancer Res.* 12: 3003-3009, 2006.
[68] Yano A, Fujii Y, Iwai A, Kawakami S, Kageyama Y, Kihara K. Glucocorticoids suppress tumor lymphangiogenesis of prostate cancer cells. *Clin. Cancer Res.* 12: 6012-6017, 2006.
[69] Wilson C, Scullin P, Worthington J, Seaton A, Maxwell P, O'Rourke D, et al. Dexamethasone potentiates the antiangiogenic activity of docetaxel in castration-resistant prostate cancer. *Br. J. Cancer.* 99: 2054-2064, 2008.
[70] Yam H. F, Wang Z. H, Or P. C, Wang S. W, Li J, Chew E. C. Effect of glucocorticoid hormone on nuclear matrix in cervical cancer cells *in vitro*. *Anticancer Res*. 18: 209-216, 1998.
[71] Samuelsson M. K. R, Pazirandeh A, Davani B, Okret S. $p57^{Kip2}$, a glucocorticoid-induced inhibitor of cell cycle progression in HeLa cells. *Mol. Endocrinol.* 13: 1811-1822, 1999.
[72] Lu Y-S, Yeh P-Y, Chuang S-E, Gao M, Kuo M-L, Cheng A-L. Glucocorticoids enhance cytotoxicity of cisplatin via suppression of NF-κB activation in the glucocorticoid receptor-rich human cervical carcinoma cell line SiHa. *J. Endocrinol.* 188: 311-319, 2006.
[73] Hayashido Y, Shirasuna K, Sugiura T, Nakashima M, Matsuya T. Effect of dexamethasone on invasion of human squamous cell carcinoma cells into collagen gel. *Cancer Lett.* 108: 81-86, 1996.
[74] Shiratsuchi T, Ishibashi H, Shirasuna K. Inhibition of epidermal growth factor-induced invasion by dexamethasone and AP-1 decoy in human squamous cell carcinoma cell lines. *J. Cell. Physiol.* 193: 340-348 2002.
[75] Shim S-H, Hah J. H, Hwang S-Y, Heo D. S, Sung M-W. Dexamethasone treatment inhibits VEGF production via suppression of STAT3 in a head and neck cancer cell line. *Oncol. Rep.* 23: 1139-1143.

[76] Murakami N, Fukuchi S, Takeuchi K, Hori T, Shibamoto S, Ito F. Antagonistic regulation of cell migration by epidermal growth factor and glucocorticoid in human gastric carcinoma cells. *J. Cell. Physiol.* 176: 127-137, 1998.

[77] Iwai A, Fujii Y, Kawakami S, Takazawa R, Kageyama Y, Yoshida M. A, et al. Down-regulation of vascular endothelial growth factor in renal cell carcinoma cells by glucocorticoids. *Mol. Cell. Endocrinol.* 226: 11-17, 2004.

[78] Arai Y, Nonomura N, Nakai Y, Nishimura K, Oka D, Shiba M, et al. The growth-inhibitory effects of dexamethasone on renal cell carcinoma *in vivo* and *in vitro. Cancer Invest.* 26: 35-40, 2008.

[79] Egberts J. H, Schniewind B, Pätzold M, Kettler B, Tepel J, Kalthoff H, et al. Dexamethasone reduces tumor recurrence and metastasis after pancreatic tumor resection in SCID mice. *Cancer Biol. Ther.* 7: 1044-1050, 2008.

[80] Evans-Storms R. B, Cidlowski J. A. Delineation of an antiapoptotic action of glucocorticoids in hepatoma cells: The role of nuclear factor-κB. *Endocrinology.* 141: 1854-1862, 2000.

[81] Dobos J, Kenessey I, Tímár J, Ladányi A. Glucocorticoid receptor expression and antiproliferative effect of dexamethasone on human melanoma cells. *Pathol. Oncol. Res.* 17: 729-734, 2011.

[82] Rogatsky, I, Trowbridge J. M, Garabedian M. J. Glucocorticoid receptor-mediated cell cycle arrest is achieved through distinct cell-specific transcriptional regulatory mechanisms. *Mol. Cell. Biol.* 17: 3181-3193, 1997.

In: Dexamethasone
Editors: A. Sauvage and M. Levy
ISBN: 978-1-62808-405-4

Chapter V

Perioperative Uses of Dexamethasone

***Ivan Parra-Sanchez*[1], *Carolina Parada*[2] *and Kenneth C. Cummings III*[1*]**
[1]Anesthesiology Institute, Cleveland Clinic, Cleveland, OH, US
[2]Lerner Research Institute, Cleveland Clinic, Cleveland, OH, US

Abstract

Dexamethasone is a synthetic glucocorticoid with an established role as an anti-inflammatory, immunosuppressant, and agent to prevent post operative nausea and vomiting. More recent evidence has demonstrated a potential role for dexamethasone in postoperative pain management, both as a systemic analgesic and adjuvant to local anesthetics for perineural use.

Dexamethasone binds to glucocorticoid receptors in the cytoplasm, dimerizes and then translocates into the nucleus. In the nucleus, it binds to specific DNA sequences to regulate gene transcription of agents involved in the function of inflammatory response mediators, such as cytokines, arachidonic acid and endothelial leukocyte adhesion molecules. Compared to other glucocorticoids, dexamethasone has the strongest anti-inflammatory effect with 30 times the potency of

* Corresponding Author Anesthesiology Institute, Cleveland Clinic, Cleveland, OH, 9500 Euclid Ave, Mailcode G30, Cleveland, OH 44195. Email: cummink2@ccf.org.

hydrocortisone. Dexamethasone has also shown to be useful in the treatment of nausea and vomiting by altering phospholipase A2 synthesis thus suppressing prostaglandin production. It is also believed that the reduction of circulating inflammatory mediators that can stimulate the chemoreceptor trigger zone in the brain may also contribute to this effect.

Moreover, a single preoperative dose of dexamethasone has shown to be an effective adjunct to reduce postoperative pain and opioid consumption after surgery. Lower pain scores might be explained by its inhibitory effect on prostaglandin production. Additionally, with the suppression of inflammatory mediators, activation of peripheral pain receptors is limited. In the same way, the use of dexamethasone with local anesthetics has been demonstrated to significantly prolong the analgesic effect of nerve blocks either by inducing vasoconstriction and thus reducing local anesthetic absorption or by increasing the activity of inhibitory potassium channels on nociceptive c-fibers, thus decreasing their activity.

Although the benefits of glucocorticoids are well known, prolonged use or high doses have significant adverse effects. Dexamethasone, as all glucocorticoids, increases levels of glucose in the blood potentially leading to glucocorticoid-induced diabetes. Extended use also can cause hypertension via renal sodium retention and potentiation of vasopressor responses to angiotensin II and catecholamines. Additionally, it reduces the proliferation of chondrocytes inducing the apoptosis of these cells thus slowing down the growth rate in children. In adults, osteoporosis and increased risk of fractures are side effects related with prolonged use. The repair and healing of aseptic wounds is also inhibited or delayed by dexamethasone, which not only blocks cytokine signaling but also inhibits the synthesis of collagen and other important factors in wound repair. Moreover, there is evidence of suppression of the hypothalamic-pituitary axis and development of glucocorticoid resistance after prolonged use of this glucocorticoid. Therefore, even though the utility of dexamethasone as an anti-inflammatory, immunosuppressive, and analgesic agent is evident, the hazards of its use must also be appreciated.

This review will summarize the evidence for the use of dexamethasone in anesthesiology and acute pain management. Molecular mechanisms (where known) will be discussed. Potential hazards and areas of uncertainty will be explored, as will future avenues of research.

Introduction

The anti-inflammatory and immune modulating effects of glucocorticoid hormones have been well established over decades. Glucocorticoids are characterized by exerting potent anti-inflammatory and immunosuppressive actions in a cell-type specific manner through the inhibition of cytokine - mediated pathways making them among the most widely prescribed drugs for the treatment of inflammatory and immune diseases. [1] Glucocorticoids also participate in other numerous physiological processes such as glucose homeostasis, blood pressure, mineral metabolism, both positive and negative effects on cell growth, and are proapoptotic. Other central effects include modulation of food intake, body temperature, pain perception, neuroendocrine function, and changes in mood and behavior. [2]A number of synthetic analogs of cortisol, the natural human glucocorticoid, have been developed and include, among others, dexamethasone.

Dexamethasone is a synthetic glucocorticoid with an established role as an anti-inflammatory, immunosuppressant, and agent to prevent postoperative nausea and vomiting. [3]More recent evidence has demonstrated a potential role for dexamethasone in postoperative pain management, both as a systemic analgesic [4] and adjuvant to local anesthetics for perineural use. [5] The aim of this review is to summarize the evidence for the use of dexamethasone in perioperative anesthesia and acute pain management as well as potential hazards and future avenues of research.

General Endogenous Glucocorticoid Mechanism of Action on Inflammation and Pain

Glucocorticoids have been widely known for their effect on the inhibition of synthesis, release, and/or efficacy of cytokines and other mediators that promote inflammatory and autoimmune reactions. The hypothalamic-pituitary-adrenal axis (HPA) plays a central role in regulating signaling via glucocorticoid receptors. [1] The central nervous system integrates a series of neural, cytokine and endocrine signals at the level of the corticotropin-releasing hormone (CRH) neurons clustered in the paraventricular hypothalamic nucleus to control the secretion of CRH into the hypophyseal portal system [2](Figure 1). Following release into the hypophyseal plexus, CRH is transported to the anterior pituitary stimulating the release of corticotropin from the anterior pituitary, which induces the secretion of cortisol by the adrenal cortex. [2] The glucocorticoid receptor (GR) is a ligand-activated transcription factor. In the absence of the ligand, it is located in the cytoplasm as a protein complex together with heat shock proteins (HSPs)-90, HSP-70 HSP-40 and other chaperone molecules. [6] GR binds with high affinity to cortisol promoting the dissociation of the HSP and molecular chaperones from the receptor facilitating ligand binding. [6,7] Within the cell, cortisol acts in three different ways (Figure 2). First, after ligand binding, the GR dissociates from its associated proteins and translocates to the nucleus interacting with specific DNA sequences called glucocorticoid response elements (GRE). The binding of the GR dimer to the GRE, called the transactivation mechanism, changes the rate of transcription, resulting in induction of genes that code for anti-inflammatory proteins such as lipocortin-1, secretory leukocyte protease inhibitors and mitogen activated protein kinase phosphatase-1. [6,7] Second, GR interacts as a monomer in the nucleus with the transcription factors of pro-inflammatory genes, such as activator protein 1 (AP1) and nuclear factor kB (NF-kB), inhibiting the activity of those transcription factors, thus, repressing the expression of the respective pro-inflammatory proteins in a mechanism of transrepression. [6-8] The third mechanism, suggests that GRs inhibit inflammation through non-genomic pathways, by inducing signaling through second messengers and membrane-associated receptors involved in activation of anti-inflammatory proteins (Figure 2). A well described non-genomic mechanism involves the activation of endothelial nitric oxide synthetase. [9]

Interactions among the hypothalamic-pituitary-adrenal axis, cytokines and inflammatory mediators play an important role on the regulation of inflammation and consequently of pain. [2] Activation of peripheral pain receptors by cytokines and inflammatory mediators carry pain signals to the dorsal horn, thalamus and somatosensory cortex, ultimately stimulating hypothalamic-pituitary-adrenal activity (Figure 1). Glucocorticoids inhibit the synthesis of cytokines and inflammatory mediators, thus causing inactivation of this nociceptive pathway. [10]

Dexamethasone, a Synthetic Glucocorticoid

Dexamethasone is an anti-inflammatory 9-fluoro-glucocorticoid that binds to glucocorticoid receptors in the cytoplasm. [1] After it dimerizes with GR it translocates into the nucleus binding then to the glucocorticoid response element resulting in induction and repression of genes related to inflammatory processes. [6,7] Dexamethasone is one of the most effective ligands for GR activation making it an effective anti-inflammatory drug.

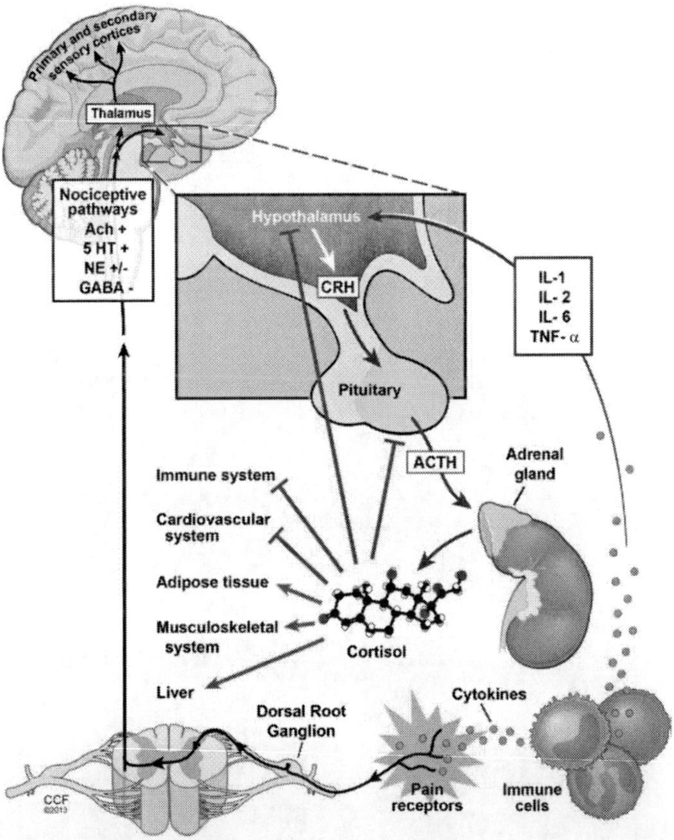

Figure 1. The Hypothalamic-Pituitary-Adrenal Axis, and Other Tissues Influenced by Immune Signals and Glucocorticoids. Cytokines and inflammatory mediators activate peripheral pain receptors, which in turn carry pain to the thalamus and somatosensory cortex via the dorsal horn of the spinal cord. Activation of these nociceptive pathways ultimately activates hypothalamic-pituitary-adrenal activity by triggering the release of CRH secretion by the hypothalamus. In turn, this signals to the pituitary to release ACTH which stimulates the adrenal gland to release cortisol. This glucocorticoid inhibits the synthesis of cytokines and inflammatory mediators, thus forming a negative feedback loop. The diagram also shows other important influences on the hypothalamic-pituitary-adrenal axis. Red lines denote inhibition, and the blue and black arrows activation.

The clinical potency of the various synthetic glucocorticoids depends on the rate of absorption, the concentration in the target tissues, the affinity for the steroid receptor, and the rate of metabolism and subsequent clearance. [11]

The main structural characteristics that determine dexamethasone's synthetic glucocorticoid potency are the size and the polarity of its substituents. It has a fluorine atom in the 9α position of ring B; a factor that increases its glucocorticoid activity when compared to other synthetic glucocorticoids [11] (Figure 3).

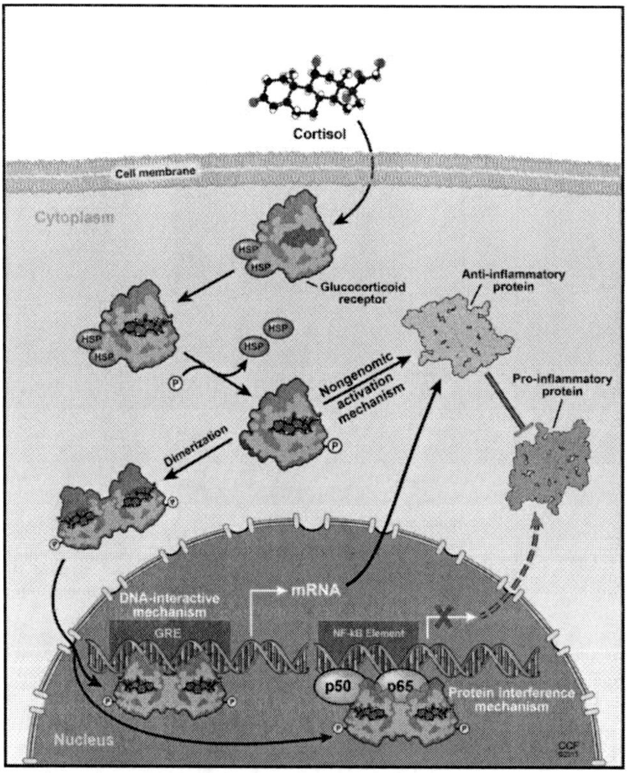

Figure 2. General Mechanisms of Action of Glucocorticoids and the Glucocorticoid Receptor in the Inhibition of Inflammation. The Glucocorticoid receptor (GR) resides in the cytoplasm complexed with several heat shock proteins (HSP). On binding to glucocorticoids, the activated receptor dissociates from the attached accessory proteins and translocates into the nucleus. The GR then regulates the expression of genes by three basic modes of action. From bottom to top: The GR physically interacts with transcription factors of pro-inflammatory genes such as factor kB (NF-kB), inhibiting the activity of those transcription factors, thus repressing the expression of the respective pro-inflammatory proteins. GR also directly interacts with specific DNA sequences called the glucocorticoid response elements (GRE) inducing the transcription of genes that code for anti-inflammatory proteins. The third mechanism, found in the cytoplasm, shows GR inflammatory inhibition by non-genomic activation. Black arrows denote activation, the red line inhibition, the red dashed arrow repression, and the red X lack of product.

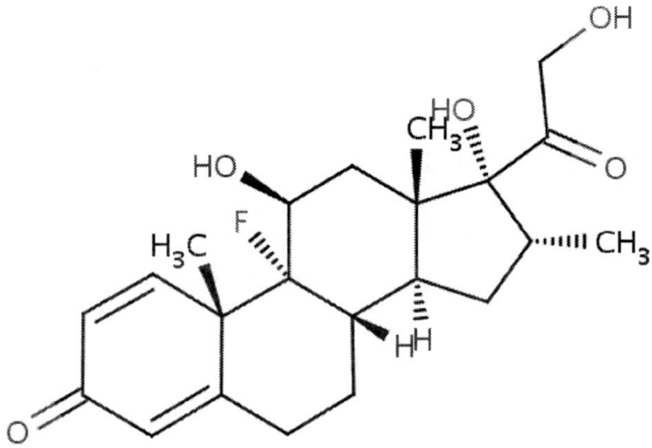

Figure 3. Chemical Structure of Dexamethasone.

Table 1. Glucocorticoid equivalencies [12,13]

Glucocorticoids	Equivalent dose (mg)	Glucocorticoid potency	Plasma half-life (min)	Biologic half-life (h)
Short-acting				
Cortisol	20.0	1.0	90	8-12
Cortisone	25.0	0.8	80-118	8-12
Intermediate-acting				
Prednisone	5.0	4.0	60	18-36
Prednisolone	5.0	5.0	115-200	18-36
Triamcinolone	4.0	5.0	30	18-36
Methylprednisolone	4.0	5.0	180	18-36
Long-acting				
Dexamethasone	0.75	30	200	36-54
Betamethasone	0.6	25-40	300	36-54

It is about 30 times more potent than cortisol and 6 times more potent than hydrocortisone. [12,13] The 9α fluorine also plays an important role in dexamethasone's metabolism; it extends dexamethasone's plasma half life to 200 minutes, and its biological half life to 36-64 hours. [12,13] Estimates of potencies of representative glucocorticoids are listed in Table 1.

Dexamethasone in the Management of Post-surgical Pain

Effective postoperative pain management is an important aspect of optimal care of surgical patients. Despite advances in the molecular understanding of inflammatory, nociceptive and stress responses, there is still a need for further improvements in postoperative pain management. A surgical operation elicits inflammatory and endocrine stress response, that when allowed to be excessive increases functional demands on various organ systems thus contributing to postoperative morbidity. [14] The use of glucocorticoids in the management of acute postoperative pain has a significant molecular basis: glucocorticoids interfere with the inflammatory process by inhibiting the release of inflammatory modulators (prostaglandins, cytokines, histamine, serotonin) and limiting the intensity and duration of pain, local hyperthermia, erythema and loss of function. [15] Glucocorticoids also suppress tissue levels of bradykinin and released neuropeptides from nerve endings which increase nociception in inflamed tissue. [16] Moreover, it has been observed that locally applied glucocorticoids inhibit the transmission of impulses in nociceptive C-fibers. [16]

The positive effects on recovery from single dose corticosteroids after pediatric tonsillectomy have been well documented. [17-19] A double-blind, placebo-controlled study in patients undergoing laparoscopic cholecystectomy observed effective pain control with the use of 8mg of preoperative dexamethasone when compared to placebo. [20] A more recent meta-analysis of twenty-four randomized clinical trials (including 2751 patients) published between 1997 and 2010 utilizing dexamethasone for postoperative pain control was conducted in 2011. [21] In the trials, 8 evaluated the use of low dose (<0.1 mg/kg) dexamethasone, 14 evaluated an intermediate dose (0.11-0.2 mg/kg) and 7 trials evaluated a high dose (>0.2 mg/kg) during different procedures (ENT, laparoscopic cholecystectomy, thyroidectomy, gynecologic surgery, breast). Each trial looked at early acute postoperative pain scores at rest and movement, and cumulative opioid consumption postoperatively. In the meta-analysis it was concluded that studies that evaluated the use of an intermediate and high dose of dexamethasone demonstrated an opioid-sparing effect and decreased early and late pain scores at rest and with movement. An important implication of these studies is that lower doses of dexamethasone given for prophylaxis against nausea and vomiting should be switched to intermediate doses to achieve the beneficial effects on postoperative pain and reduction of opioid consumption. [21] Moreover, the high dose dexamethasone group showed a reduction in late pain at movement compared with the intermediate dose group, but did not show a significant advantage in the opioid usage. When evaluating early pain at rest, 3 groups using high to intermediate doses of dexamethasone showed decrease in early pain at rest but the low dose group did not show a statistically significant reduction. [21]

The most recent meta-analysis [4] included forty-five randomized, controlled studies involving 5796 patients who received single perioperative doses of dexamethasone between 1.25 to 20 mg compared with placebo and another antiemetic agent. The authors analyzed reported pain scores, analgesic consumption, rescue analgesics and time to first dose of analgesics. Patients treated with dexamethasone experienced less postoperative pain, required less postoperative opioids, had longer time to first analgesic use, needed less rescue analgesia, and had shorter PACU stays. [4] Patients having laparoscopic surgery did not have any difference in opioid consumption as compared with open abdominal surgery which showed a 3 mg morphine reduction in the first 24 hours. The authors concluded that even though the analgesic effects of a single-dose of dexamethasone were statistically significant, they were small and not clinically relevant. [4]

The downsides observed in the previous meta-analysis include lack of limitation of evaluation of dexamethasone in which pain is the primary outcome, because most of the trials evaluated postoperative nausea and vomiting as the primary outcome. Therefore, the variability in the type of surgery added to dexamethasone dose and timing, as well as anesthetic regimen should be factors that need to be controlled in further studies evaluating the use of single dose dexamethasone. Moreover, there is a need for larger randomized controlled trials using dexamethasone in which pain is the primary outcome. Even though, there is increasing evidence about the positive effects of a single dose of dexamethasone as a part of postoperative pain control management, currently dexamethasone in not being used as a component of a multimodal drug strategy to treat postoperative pain [21]probably to the lack of strong evidence observed in the different studies.

Dexamethasone and Regional Anesthesia

The prolongation of surgical anesthesia and analgesia has been of significant interest in regional anesthesia. In order to increase the duration of local anesthetic action and improve the quality of nerve blocks, investigators have used different adjuvant drugs mixed with local anesthetics. Adjuvants such as epinephrine, clonidine, [22,23] ketamine, [24,25] opioids, [26,27] midazolam [28] and glucocorticoids (dexamethasone) [29-34] have been used in different studies with high quality outcomes.

Why glucocorticoids and in this case dexamethasone prolong the effect of nerve blocks is still under discussion. [35] Three studies have observed that corticosteroids substantially reduce the stimulus transmission in unmyelinated C-fibers, known to carry mainly nociceptive information by inhibiting the activity of potassium channels on these fibers. [35,36,37]

Other mechanisms involve certain degree of vasoconstriction caused by glucocorticoids which reduces the local absorption increasing duration of local anesthetics. Also, the potent anti-inflammatory effect of glucocorticoids has been shown to inhibit the release of inflammatory mediators (interleukins, cytokines, etc), and facilitate the release of anti-inflammatory mediators thus decreasing postoperative pain. [15]

Parrington and colleagues [32] added 8 mg of dexamethasone to 1.5% mepivacaine for ultrasound-guided supraclavicular blocks and concluded a statistically significant prolongation of the duration of analgesia (median 332 min) compared to mepivacaine with normal saline (median 228 min). The patients in the dexamethasone group had significantly reduced opioid requirements in PACU and significantly reduced pain scores at 8 hours postoperatively. Vieira et al. [34] showed a significant increase in the median sensory duration (1457 vs. 833 min) of ultrasound-guided interscalene blocks when dexamethasone (8 mg) was added to 0.5% bupivacaine, epinephrine and clonidine as compared to the same components without dexamethasone. This is approximately a 12 hour longer duration of analgesia along with a decrease in postoperative opioid usage.

Furthermore, Tandoc and colleagues [38] reported that both doses 4 mg and 8 mg of dexamethasone mixed with 0.5% bupivacaine were similarly effective at prolonging the duration of interscalene nerve blocks in patients undergoing shoulder surgery. They also showed a decrease in opioid consumption in the first 48 hours postoperatively. Kim et al. [39] used a 5mg dose of dexamethasone combined with 0.5% levobupivacaine in ultrasound guided interscalene blocks for arthroscopic shoulder surgery. They showed excellent extension of the block and pain scores notably lower than when adding normal saline or epinephrine to the local anesthetic. No complications or side effects were reported. Movafegh et al. [31] published a study on the effect of dexamethasone in axillary nerve blocks. The authors concluded that by adding 8 mg of dexamethasone to 1.5% lidocaine prolonged the duration of the sensory block from 98 to 242 minutes.

Moreover, Cummings, et al. [5] published the first study to examine the effect of dexamethasone on ropivacaine for interscalene nerve blocks and the largest randomized trial to date to study the outcomes of using adjuvant dexamethasone in peripheral nerve blocks. This study showed a marked (from 11.8 to 22.2 hrs and from 14.8 to 22.4 hrs) increase in block duration when adding 8 mg of dexamethasone to ropivacaine and bupivacaine, respectively, as compared to plain ropivacaine and bupivacaine.

In conclusion, previous studies have demonstrated that dexamethasone prolongs the duration of different peripheral nerve blocks with the use of a variety of local anesthetics. It is difficult to compare the different studies performed to date because of the different blocks used, different kinds of local anesthetics used and different methods to assess the duration of the different blocks performed. Furthermore, concerns about safety for the use of dexamethasone in peripheral nerve blocks due to possible neurotoxicity have been cited. [31] No trial to date has reported neurotoxicity related to the utilization of dexamethasone for peripheral nerve blocks. However, it is well known that local anesthetics can be neurotoxic. Recently, Ma et al. [40] showed a protective effect of dexamethasone on mice neurons that had been exposed to bupivacaine and lidocaine. The authors suggest that pretreatment of neuroblastoma cells with dexamethasone exerts a protective effect on bupivacaine and lidocaine-induced neuronal cell injury. Ultimately, however, larger scale studies have to be performed to be able to detect uncommon complications.

Dexamethasone in the Prevention of Postoperative Nausea and Vomiting

Postoperative nausea and vomiting (PONV) is one of the leading causes for delayed discharge and unplanned hospital admissions following outpatient surgery. [41] These factors continue to be significant problems following anesthesia. Anesthetics and opioids stimulate the chemoreceptor trigger zone and the brain stem vomiting center, which are modulated by serotonin (5-HT), histamine, acetylcholine, and dopamine. [42] Dexamethasone has shown to be useful in the treatment of postoperative nausea and vomiting probably by altering phospholipase A_2 synthesis thus suppressing prostaglandin production.

[1,43] It is also believed that the reduction of circulating inflammatory mediators that can stimulate the chemoreceptor trigger zone in the brain may also contribute to this effect by inhibiting prostaglandin synthesis or inhibiting the release of endogenous opioids. [43,44] Moreover, it has been suggested that the control of emesis might be caused by the release of endorphins, resulting in mood elevation, a sense of well-being and appetite stimulation. [44]

Even though the exact mechanism of action of dexamethasone in the prevention of PONV is not yet well understood, the use of single-dose dexamethasone in the prevention of PONV has been well established. The first clinical trial that suggested that dexamethasone may prevent PONV was published in 1993. [45] Later studies have been conducted indicating that dexamethasone is indeed a good alternative for the control of nausea and vomiting symptoms in the postoperative period. In a meta-analysis of seventeen randomized controlled trials with data from 1,946 subjects evaluating the use of dexamethasone as a single prophylactic dose to treat POVN it was found that dexamethasone alone or in combination with a 5-HT3 receptor antagonist was effective in the control of postoperative emetic symptoms. [46] A single dose of dexamethasone markedly reduced PONV when compared to placebo in seven trials (4 adult and 3 children). [46-48] Experimental results have also shown an increased anti-emetic effect of dexamethasone when added to a 5-HT3 receptor antagonist. Fourteen randomized control trials evaluated the effect of dexamethasone treatment combined with a 5-HT3 receptor antagonist (ondansetron, granisetron, or tropisetron) versus a 5-HT3 receptor antagonist alone on PONV. The results showed decreased PONV when dexamethasone was used in combination with a 5-HT3 receptor antagonist. [48-61] The reasons that can explain the effectiveness of this combined therapy may be attributed first to the effect that glucocorticoids have on reducing the levels of 5-hydroxytryptamine type 3 receptors in neural tissue, [62] and second, to the anti-inflammatory properties of glucocorticoids preventing the release of serotonin in the gut. [63]

Current recommendations from the Society of Ambulatory Anesthesia (SAMBA) for the management of PONV include a 4-mg to 5-mg dose regimen of systemic dexamethasone. [64] Patients at low risk for PONV are usually not given PONV prophylaxis unless they are at risk for medical complications from vomiting (i.e., patients with high intracranial pressure or who are having fundoplication surgery). [65] Current guidelines only recommend prophylactic PONV treatment for those patients at moderate to high risk for PONV. Table 2 contains the risk factors reported by SAMBA for

PONV in adults. [65] Moreover, different studies have observed greater effectiveness of dexamethasone in the prophylactic treatment of PONV when administered before the induction of anesthesia rather than at the end. [66]

Table 2. Risk Factors for Postoperative Nausea and Vomiting (PONV) in Adults [64]

<table>
<tr><td>Patient-specific risk factors</td><td>Patient-specific risk factors</td><td>Surgical risk factors</td></tr>
<tr><td>Female gender</td><td>Use of volatile anesthetics</td><td rowspan="2">Duration of surgery: Each 30-min increase in duration increases PONV risk by 60%, so that a baseline risk of 10% is increased by 16% after 30 min.</td></tr>
<tr><td>Nonsmoking status</td><td>Nitrous oxide systematic review</td></tr>
<tr><td>History of PONV/motion sickness.</td><td>Use of intraoperative and postoperative opioids</td><td>Type of surgery: Laparoscopy, laparotomy, breast, strabismus, plastic surgery, maxillofacial, gynecological, abdominal, neurologic, ophthalmologic and urologic</td></tr>
</table>

Adverse Effects of a Single Dose Dexamethasone in the Perioperative Treatment of Pain and PONV

The benefits of glucocorticoids are well established remaining an important component of therapy for many conditions. Their clinical success as effective anti-inflammatory agents is attributed to their ability to reduce the expression of proinflammatory genes and the inhibition of the activity of proinflammatory transcription factors. [6] In spite of this, their clinical use is compromised by related adverse effects specially when used for prolonged periods of time or used at high doses (>0.2mg/kg). [67] These side effects are largely related to glucocorticoid receptor's ability to activate target genes involved in the metabolism of sugar, fat, proteins, muscle and bone. [6,67] Examples of different conditions related to prolonged or high dose usage of glucocorticoids include: dyslipidemia, hypertension, thrombosis, adrenal atrophy, pancreatitis, peptic ulcer, broad immunosuppression, delayed wound healing, erythema, osteoporosis, muscle atrophy, retardation of longitudinal long bone growth, glaucoma, and delayed puberty among others. [67] Short term use of glucocorticoids, on the other hand, is characterized by short-term vascular changes and limited immunosuppression, [67] thus making them an appealing type of treatment for acute pain control and postoperative nausea and vomiting during perioperative therapy.

In a meta-analysis published in 2013 evaluating the impact of perioperative single dose systemic dexamethasone for postoperative pain, patients treated with dexamethasone did not demonstrate a significantly increased risk of infection or wound healing. [4] Fourteen studies (1449 patients) examined the incidence of wound infection. From those, eleven found no reported infection related to the use of dexamethasone or use of placebo in treated patients. In the three remaining studies (235 patients), there was no increase of infection in patients receiving dexamethasone. Nine studies (1020 patients) examining the incidence of wound healing found no difference in either dexamethasone-treated or placebo-treated patients. [4] Therefore, even though it is well known that glucocorticoid-mediated effects are multifactorial and prevent the early inflammatory phase, which is essential for efficient wound repair; [1] a single perioperative dose of dexamethasone, as opposed to long term use, has not been associated with delayed wound healing and increased risk of infection. [4,21]

A potential limitation to the use of dexamethasone in perioperative therapy is the incidence of perineal pruritus when given rapidly in low volumes. The first reported case was in 2003 [68] following intravenous administration of dexamethasone before general anesthesia to prevent postoperative nausea and vomiting in three consecutive surgical patients. The authors subsequently conducted a study to evaluate the incidence of dexamethasone-induced perineal pruritus in 20 surgical patients (10 males and 10 females), and concluded that female patients seem more at risk of this complication. [68] Another study reported two cases of unexpected perineal pain immediately after intravenous injection of fentanyl and dexamethasone during induction of general anesthesia. In both cases, the pain was immediate (onset within 30 seconds), severe, localized to the genital region and of shooting and burning character. [69] The exact mechanism by which dexamethasone induces perineal pruritus is unknown, but it can frequently (50-70%) produce extreme perineal pain. [21]

Limitations of single dose perioperative dexamethasone therapy also include elevation of blood glucose levels. Glucocorticoids in the periphery diminish glucose utilization, increase protein break down and activate lipolysis, as a mechanism of protection of glucose-dependent tissues from starvation. A single perioperative dose of dexamethasone has shown to elevate intraoperative blood glucose for 4 hours. [70] Two studies measured perioperative blood glucose in non-diabetic patients observing small but statistically significant elevations in blood glucose levels at 24 hours after operation, [71,72] thus demonstrating that blood glucose levels elevation extends for 24 hours. Studies have reported an association of blood glucose elevation with high BMI and high baseline HBA1c. [73] The use of dexamethasone or other types of corticosteroid therapy have not been associated with any postoperative complication related to increased glucose levels; therefore, there are not current limitations in the use of single dose dexamethasone for the treatment of pain and PONV in non-cardiac patients. On the other hand, poor intraoperative control of blood glucose levels is known to adversely affect patient outcome after cardiac surgery. In a study evaluating two hundred patients undergoing heart surgery, poor intraoperative glycemic control (four consecutive blood glucose levels higher than 200mg/dL) was associated with severe cardiovascular, respiratory, infectious, neurologic, and renal in-hospital morbidity. [74]

Future Directions

Today, the most important limiting factors in the use of glucocorticoids are its side effects. Therefore, there is a strong need to develop compounds with the anti-inflammatory potency of present synthetic glucocorticoids but with fewer side effects. A number of side effects seem to be mediated by a transactivation mechanism, in which the glucocorticoid receptor (GR) binds to DNA activating genes that code for anti-inflammatory proteins. [75] Consequently, an innovative therapy would consist in the identification of glucocorticoids that would prefer GR-protein interaction instead of GR-DNA interaction. Recently, a novel class of steroids (RU24858, RU4006, RU40066, ZK245186 and ZK216348) has demonstrated a dissociated effect with potent transrepression activity and weak transactivation activity, thus suggesting that development of steroids with specific selectivity might reduce adverse effects associated with the use of glucocorticoids. [76]

Moreover, deeper understanding on glucocorticoid action needs to be further explored, due to recent findings showing that the response pattern of glucocorticoids is gene dependent within one cell type, and fluctuates from slowly and continuous to transiently and rapid, and sustained repression. [77] Consequently, optimization of the pharmacodynamics and pharmacokinetics of new drugs are also important tasks for the near future.

References

[1] Schimmer BP, Parker K. Adrenocorticotropic hormone; adrenocortical steroids and their synthetic analogs; inhibitors of the synthesis and actions of adrenocortical hormones. In: Brunton L, Chabner B (eds). *Goodman and Gilman's: The Pharmacological Basis of Therapeutics,* 10th edition, McGraw-Hill Medical; 2001: Chapter 59.

[2] Turnbull AV, Rivier CL. Regulation of the Hypothalamic-pituitary-adrenal axis by cytokines: actions and mechanisms of action. *Physiological Reviews* 1999;79:1-71.

[3] De Oliveira GS, Santana L, Ahmad S, Kendall M, McCarthy R. Dexamethasone to prevent post operative nausea and vomiting: An updated meta-analysis of randomized control trials. *Society for Ambulatory Anesthesiology* 2013;116:58-74.

[4] Waldron NH, Jones CA, Gan TJ, Allen TK, Habib AS. Impact of perioperative dexamethasone on postoperative analgesia and side effects: systematic review and meta-analysis. *Br J Anaesth* 2013; 110(2): 191-200.

[5] Cummings III KC, Napierkowski DE, Parra-Sanchez I, Kurz A, Dalton JE, Brems JJ, Sessler DI. Effect of dexamethasone on the duration of interscalene nerve block with ropivacaine and bupivacaine. *Br J Anaesth* 2011; 107(3): 446-53.

[6] Barnes PJ. Anti-inflammatory actions of glucocorticoids: molecular mechanisms. *Clinical Science.* 1998;94:557-572.

[7] Sapolsky RM, Romero M, Munck A. How do Glucocorticoid influence stress responses? Integrating permissive, stimulatory and preparative actions. *Endocrine Reviews* 2000;21(1):55-89.

[8] Barnes PJ, Karin M. Nuclear Factor-KB: A pivotal transcription factor in chronic inflammatory diseases. *1997 N Engl J Med* 336:1066-71.

[9] Hafezi-Moghadam A, Simoncini T, Yanz Z, et al. Acute Cardiovascular protective effects of corticoesteroids are mediated by non transcriptional activation of endothelial nitric oxide synthase. *Nat Med* 2002;8:473-9.

[10] Rivest S. How Circulating cytokines trigger the neural circuits that control the hypothalamic-pituitary-adrenal axis. *Psycho-neuroendocrinology* 2001; 26:761-88.

[11] Diederich S, Eigendorff E, Burkhardt P, Quinkler M, Bumke-Vogt C, Rochel M, Seidelmann D, Esperling P, Oelkers W, Bhr V. 11beta-hydroxysteroid dehydrogenase types 1 and 2: an important pharmacokinetic determinant for the activity of synthetic mineralo and glucocorticoids. *J Clin Endocrinol Metab.* 2002;87(12):5695-701.

[12] Chrousos GP. *Adrenocorticosteroids & Adrenocortical Antagonists.* In: Bertram G Katzung (ed) Basic & Clinical Pharmacology, tenth edition, McGraw-Hill Medical; 2007: Chapter 3.

[13] Stewart PM. The adrenal cortex. In: Kronenberg HM, Melmed S, Polonsky KS, Larsen RP (eds). *Williams Textbook of Endocrinology,* 11th edition, Saunders; 2008: Chapter 14.

[14] Wilmore DW. Metabolic response to severe surgical illness: Overview. *World J Surg* 2000;24:705-711.

[15] Troullos ES, Hargraves KM, Butler DP, Dionne RA: Comparison of nonsteroidal anti-inflammatory drugs, ibuprofen and flurbiprofen, with methylprednisolone and placebo for acute pain, swelling and trismus. *J Oral Maxillofac Surg* 1990; 48: 945-952.

[16] Holte K, Kehlet H. Perioperative single-dose glucocorticoid administration: Pathophysiologic effects and clinical implications. *J Am Coll Surg* 2002; 195: 694-712.

[17] Goldman AC, Govindaraj S, Rosenfeld RM. A meta-analysis of dexamethasone use with tonsillectomy. *Otolaryngol Head Neck Surg* 2000; 123:682– 686.

[18] Windfuhr JP. *Steroids for reduction of morbidity following tonsillectomy.* HNO 2008; 56:43–53.

[19] Steward DL, Welge JA, Myer CM. Steroids for improving recovery following tonsillectomy in children. *Cochrane Database Syst Rev* 2003: CD003997.

[20] Bisgaard T, Klarskov B, Kehlet H, Rosenberg J. Preoperative dexamethasone improves surgical outcome after laparoscopic cholecystectomy: a randomized double-blind placebo-controlled trial. *Ann Surg* 2003; 238:651–660.

[21] De Oliveira GS, Almeida MD, Benzon HT, McCarthy RJ. Perioperative single dose systemic dexamethasone for postoperative pain. *Anesthesiology* 2011; 115: 575-88.

[22] Andan T, Elif AA, Ayse K, Gulnaz A. Clonidine as an adjuvant for lidocaine in axillary brachial plexus block in patients with chronic renal failure. *Acta Anaesthesiol Scand* 2005; 49: 563-8.

[23] Duma A, Urbanek B, Sitzwohl C, Zimpfer M, Kapral S. Clonidine as an adjuvant to local anaesthetic axillary brachial plexus block: a randomized, controlled study. *Br J Anaesth* 2005; 94: 112–6.

[24] Clerc S, Vuillermier H, Frascarolo P, Spahn DR, Gardaz J. Is the effect of inguinal field block with 0.5% bupivacaine on postoperative pain after hernia repair enhanced by addition of ketorolac or S(+) ketamine? *Clin J Pain* 2005; 21: 101–5.

[25] Noyan A. On effects of ketamine to axillary block in hand surgery. *J Reconstr Microsurg* 2002; 18: 197.

[26] Karakaya D, Buyukgoz F, Baris S, Guldogus F, Tur A. Addition of fentanyl to bupivacaine prolongs anesthesia and analgesia in axillary brachial plexus block. *Reg Anesth Pain Med* 2001; 26: 434–8.

[27] Fanelli G, Casati A, Magistris L, et al. Fentanyl does not improve the nerve block characteristics of axillary brachial plexus anesthesia performed with ropivacaine. *Acta Anaesthesiol Scand* 2001; 45: 590–4.

[28] Jarbo K, Batra YK, Panda NB. Brachial plexus block with midazolam and bupivacaine improves analgesia. *Can J Anaesth* 2005; 52: 822–6.

[29] Colombo G, Padera R, Langer R, Kohane DS. Prolonged duration local anesthesia with lipid-protein-sugar particles containing bupivacaine and dexamethasone. *J Biomed Mater Res* A 2005; 75: 458–64.

[30] Drager C, Benziger D, Gao F, Berde CB. Prolonged intercostal nerve blockade in sheep using controlled-release of bupivacaine and dexamethasone from polymer microspheres. *Anesthesiology* 1998; 89: 969–79.

[31] Movafegh A, Razazian M, Hajimaohamadi F, Meysamie A. Dexamethasone added to lidocaine prolongs axillary brachial plexus blockade. *Anesth Analg* 2006; 102: 263–7.

[32] Parrington SJ, O'Donnell D, Chan VWS, et al. Dexamethasone added to mepivacaine prolongs the duration of analgesia after supraclavicular brachial plexus blockade. *Reg Anesth Pain Med* 2010; 35: 422–6.

[33] Shrestha BR, Maharjan SK, Tabedar S. Supraclavicular brachial plexus block with and without dexamethasone—a comparative study. *Kathmandu Univ Med J* 2003; 1: 158–60.

[34] Vieira PA, Pulai I, Tsao GC, Manikantan P, Keller B, Connelly NR.Dexamethasone with bupivacaine increases duration of analgesia in ultrasound-guided interscalene brachial plexus blockade. *Eur J Anaesthesiol* 2010; 27: 285–8.

[35] Johansson A, Hao J, Sjolund B. *Local corticosteroid application blocks transmission in normal nociceptive C-fibers* 1990: 34; 335-338.

[36] Attari B, Takimoto K, Gealy R, Severns C, Levitan ES. Glucocorticoid induced up-regulation of a pituitary K+ channel mRNA in vitro and in vivo. *Receptors Channels* 1993; 1: 287-93.

[37] Kopacz DJ, Lacouture PG, Wu D, Nandy P, Swanton R, Landau C. The dose response and effects of dexamethasone on bupivacaine microcapsules for intercostal blockade (T9 to T11) in healthy volunteers. *Anesth Analg* 2003; 96: 576-82.

[38] Tandoc MN, Fan L, Kolesnikov S, Kruglov A, Nader ND. Adjuvant dexamethasone with bupivacaine prolongs the duration of interscalene block: a prospective randomized trial. *J Anesth* 2011; 25(5): 704-9.

[39] Kim YG, Lee GY, Kim CH, Baik HJ, Heo S. Dexamethasone added to levobupivacaine improves postoperative analgesia in ultrasound guided interscalene brachial plexus blockade for arthroscopic shoulder surgery. *Korean J Anesthesiol* 2012; 62(2): 130-4.

[40] Ma R, Wang X, Lu C, Cheng Y, Ding G, Liu L, Ding Z. Dexamethasone attenuated bupivacaine-induced neuron injury in vitro through a threonine-serine protein kinase B-dependent mechanism. *2010 Neuroscience;* 167: 329-342.

[41] Parra-Sanchez I, Abdallah R, You J, Fu AZ, Grady Martin, Cummings III K, Apfel C, Sessler D. A time-motion economic analysis of postoperative nausea and vomiting in ambulatory surgery. *Canadian Journal of Anesthesia* 2012;59:366-375.

[42] Watcha M, White P. Postoperative Nausea and Vomiting: Its Ethiology, Treatment, and Prevention. *Anesthesiology* 1992; 77:162-184.

[43] Rich W, Abdulhayoglu G, Di Saia PJ. Methylprednisolone as antiemetic during cancer chemotherapy: a pilot study. *Gynecol Oncol* 1980; 9:193-8.

[44] Harris AL. Cytotoxic-therapy-induced vomiting is mediated via enkephalin pathways. *Lancet* 1982;1:714-6.

[45] Baxendale BR, VAter M, Lavery KM. Dexamethasoe reduces pain and swelling following extraction of third molar teeth. *Anesthesia* 1993;48:961-4.

[46] Henzi I, Walder B, Tramer MT. Dexamethasone for the prevention of postoperative nausea and vomiting: A quantitative systematic review. *Anesthesia Analg* 2000;90:186-94.
[47] Liu K, Hsu CC, Chia YY. Effect of dexamethasone on postoperative emesis and pain. *Br J Anaesth* 1998;80:85–6.
[48] Fujii Y, Tanaka H, Toyooka H. The effects of dexamethasone on antiemetics in female patients undergoing gynecologic surgery. *Anesth* Analg 1997;85:913–7.
[49] Rothenberg DM, McCarthy RJ, Peng CC, Normoyle DA. Nausea and vomiting after dexamethasone versus droperidol following outpatient laparoscopy with a propofol-based general anesthetic. *Acta Anaesthesiol Scand* 1998;42:637– 42.
[50] McKenzie R, Riley TJ, Tantisira B, Hamilton DL. Effect of propofol for induction and ondansetron with or without dexamethasone for the prevention of nausea and vomiting after major gynecologic surgery. *J Clin Anesth* 1997;9:15–20.
[51] Lopez-Olaondo L, Carrascosa F, Pueyo FJ, et al. Combination of ondansetron and dexamethasone in the prophylaxis of postop- erative nausea and vomiting. *Br J Anaesth* 1996;76:835–40.
[52] Fujii Y, Tanaka H, Toyooka H. Granisetron-dexamethasone combination reduces postoperative nausea and vomiting. *Can J Anaesth* 1995;42:387–90.
[53] McKenzie R, Tantisira B, Karambelkar DJ, et al. Comparison of ondansetron with ondansetron plus dexamethasone in the prevention of postoperative nausea and vomiting. *Anesth Analg* 1994;79:961– 4.
[54] De Oliveira GS, Santana L, Ahmad S, Kendall M, McCarthy R. Dexamethasone to prevent post operative nausea and vomiting: An updated meta-analysis of randomized control trials. *Society for Ambulatory Anesthesiology* 2013;116:58-74.
[55] Fujii Y, Tanaka H, Toyooka H. Granisetron and dexamethasone provide more improved prevention of postoperative emesis than granisetron alone in children. *Can J Anaesth* 1996;43: 1229 –32.
[56] Fujii Y, Toyooka H, Tanaka H. Prophylactic antiemetic therapy with a combination of granisetron and dexamethasone in patients undergoing middle ear surgery. *Br J Anaesth* 1998;81: 754–6.
[57] Rajeeva V, Bhardwaj N, Batra YK, Dhaliwal LK. Comparison of ondasetron with ondansetron and dexamethasone in prevention of PONV in diagnostic laparoscopy. *Canadian J Anesth* 1999; 46:40-44.

[58] Karanicolas PJ, Smith SE, Kanbur B, Davies E, Guyatt GH. The impact of prophylactic dexamethasone on nausea and vomiting after laparoscopic cholecystectomy:a systematic review and meta-analysis. *Ann Surg* 2008; 248:751-62.

[59] Arslan M, Demir ME. Prevention of postoperative nausea and vomiting with a small dose of propofol combined with dexamethasone 4mg or dexamethasone 8mg in patients undergoing middle ear surgery: a prospective randomized, double-blind study. *Bratisl Lek Listy* 2011;112:332-6.

[60] D'souza N, Swami M, Bagwat S. Comparative study of dexamethasone and ondansetron for prophylaxis of postoperative nausea and vomiting laparoscopic gynecologic surgery. *Int J Gynaecol Obstet* 2011;113:124-7.

[61] Pan PH, Lee SC, Harris LC. Antiemetic prophylaxis for post discharge nausea and vomiting in and impact of functional quality of living during recovery in patients with high emetic risks:a prospective, randomized, double-blind comparison of two prophylactic antiemetic regimens. *Anesth Analg* 2008; 107:429-38.

[62] Young S. Mechanism of decline in rat brain 5-hydroxytryptamine after induction of liver tryptophan pyrrolase by hydrocortisone: roles of tryptophane catabolism and kynurenine synthesis. *Br J Pharmacol* 1981;74:695.

[63] Frederikson M, Hursti T, Fu¨rst C, et al. Nausea in cancer chemotherapy is inversely related to urinary cortisol excretion. *Br J Cancer* 1992;65:779–80.

[64] Gan TJ, Meyer TA, Apfel CC, Chung F, Davis PJ, Habib AS, Hooper VD, Kovac AL, Kranke P, Myles P, Philip BK, Smasa G, Sessler DI, Temo J, Tramer MR, Vander Kolk C, Watcha M. Society for Ambulatory Anesthesia guidelines for the management of postoperative nausea and vomiting. *Anesth Analg* 2007;105:1615-28.

[65] Apfel CC, Kranke P, Eberhart LH, et al. Comparison of predictive models for postoperative nausea and vomiting. *Br J Anaesth* 2002;88:234–40.

[66] Wang JJ, Ho ST, Tzeng JI, Tang CS. The effect of timing of dexamethasone administration on its efficacy as a prophylactic antiemetic for postoperative nausea and vomiting. *Anesth Analg* 2000;91:136–9.

[67] Schacke H, Docke W, Asadullah K. Mechanisms involved in the side effects of glucocorticoids. *Pharmacology and Therapeutics* 2010;96:23-43.

[68] Perron G, Dolbec P, Germain J, Béchard P. Perineal pruritus after iv dexamethasone administration. *Canadian Journal of Anaesthesia* 2003; 50: 749–50.

[69] Neff SPW, Stapelberg F, Warmington A. Excruciating perineal pain after intravenous dexamethasone. *Anaesthesia and Intensive Care,* 2002;30:370-371.

[70] Pasternak JJ, McGregor DG, Lanier WL. Effect of single dose dexamethasone on blood glucose concentration in patients undergoing craniotomy. *J Neurosurg Anesthesiol* 2004;16:122-5.

[71] Feroci F, Rettori M, Borrelli A, Lenzi E, Ottaviano A, Scatizzi M. Dexamethasone prophylaxis before thyroidectomy to reduce postoperative nausea, pain and vocal dysfunction: a randomized clinical controlled trial. *Head Neck* 2011: 33:840-6.

[72] Feo CV, , Sortini D, Ragazzi R, De Palma M, Liboni A. Randomized clinical trial of the effect of preoperative dexamethasone on nausea and vomiting after laparoscopic cholecystectomy. *Br J Surg* 2006; 93:295-9.

[73] Hans P, Vanthuyne A, Dewandre PY, Brichant JF, Bonhomme V. Blood glucose concentration profile after 10mg dexamethasone in non-diabetic and type 2 diabetic patients undergoing abdominal surgery. *Br J Anaesth* 2006; 97:164-70.

[74] Ouattara A, Lecompte P, Le Manach Y, Landi M, Jacqueminet S, Platonov I, Bonnet, N, Riou B, Coriat P. Poor intraopertavie blood glucose control is associated with a worsened hospital outcome after cardiac surgey in diabetic patients. *Anesthesiology* 2005; 103(4): 687-694.

[75] Newton R. Molecular mechanisms of glucocorticoid action:what is important?. *Thorax* 2000; 55: 603-613.

[76] Strehl C, Buttgereit F. Optimized glucocorticoid therapy: Teaching old drugs new tricks. *Molecualr and Cellular Endocrinology* (2013).http://dx.doi.org/10.1016/j.mce.2013.01.026.

[77] John S, Johnson TA, Sung MH, Biddie SC, Trump S, Koch-Paiz CA, Davis SR, Walker R, Meltzer PS, Hager GL. Kinetic complexity of the global response due to glucocorticoid receptor action. *Endocrinology* 2009; 150:1776-1774.

In: Dexamethasone
Editors: A. Sauvage and M. Levy
ISBN: 978-1-62808-405-4

Chapter VI

Comparison between Cortisol's and Dexamethasone's Negative Feedback Action in Humans: Evidence for Preferential Sensitivity to the Natural Glucocorticoid

Roberta Giordano[1*], Valentina D'Angelo, Clizia Zichi, Federica Guaraldi, Marco Minetto, Ezio Ghigo, and Emanuela Arvat

[1]Department of Biological and Clinical Sciences,
Division of Endocrinology, Diabetology and Metabolism,
Department of Medical Sciences,
University of Turin, Italy

* Correspondence: Roberta Giordano, MD, Division of Endocrinology, Diabetology and Metabolism, Department of Medical Sciences, C. Dogliotti 14, 10126 Turin, ITALY. Tel: +39.011/6709586, Fax: +39.011/6647421; E-mail: roberta.giordano@unito.it.

Abstract

Glucocorticoids (GCs) inhibit HPA axis through different mechanisms and target sites mediated by two receptor types (glucocorticoid receptor, GR, and mineralcorticoid receptor, MR). Within the brain, GRs are mostly distributed in the hypothalamus and in the pituitary, and bind both natural and synthetic GCs; MRs are mainly located in the limbic structures where show high affinity for GCs. HPA response to GCs feedback is usually tested by dexamethasone, a synthetic GC that poorly penetrates BBB and preferentially activates pituitaric GRs. Differently from dexamethasone, cortisol could better evaluate the GC feedback action by acting also at supra-pituitary level. We studied the effects of different doses of hydrocortisone (HC, 15, 30 or 60 μg/kg/h, infused for 150 min) or dexamethasone (DEX, 0.4, 0.8 or 1.6 μg/kg/h, infused for 150 min) on ACTH and cortisol levels in 6 normal subjects (NS, age 25±2.1 yr, BMI 23.0±1.2 kg/m^2). The effects of HC and DEX were compared with those of placebo. Blood samples were taken every 15 min for 240 min. During placebo, ACTH and cortisol levels showed progressive decrease (baseline vs nadir, mean±SEM: 17.6±1.6 vs 13.4±0.7 pg/ml and 157.6±25.6 vs 71.7±10.6 μg/l, $p<0.05$). The dose of 15 μg/kg/h HC mantained constant cortisol but did not modify ACTH levels at any time. The doses of 30 and 60 μg/kg/h HC induced dose-dependent cortisol increases (peaks, 30 μg/kg/h: 170.5±14.8 μg/l, $p<0.05$; 60 μg/kg/h: 203.2±26.6 μg/l, $p<0.05$) associated to dose-dependent ACTH decrease (nadir, 30 μg/kg/h: 8.1±0.9 pg/ml, $p<0.05$; 60 μg/kg/h: 7.9±0.7 pg/ml, $p<0.05$). DEX at doses of 0.4, 0.8 and 1.6 μg/kg/h did not modify cortisol levels at any time. Only 1.6 μg/kg/h DEX induced an ACTH decrease ($p<0.05$) more pronounced than that after placebo (8.0±3.1 pg/ml) while neither 0.4 nor 0.8 μg/kg/h affected ACTH levels at any time. In conclusion, taking into account the potency at the GR level, doses of dexamethasone relatively higher than hydrocortisone are needed to inhibit ACTH secretion in humans. These findings are likely to reflect different sites where natural and synthetic GCs exert their feedback action, i.e. mainly the CNS for cortisol and the pituitary for dexamethasone. It is suggested that the HPA sensitivity to the feedback action of GCs in various pathophysiological conditions would better be evaluated by using natural GCs.

Keywords: Feedback, ACTH, cortisol, dexamethasone, humans

Introduction

The activity of the hypothalamus-pituitary-adrenal (HPA) axis is mainly regulated by the hypothalamic neurohormones CRH and AVP which are, in turn, under the influence of several neurotransmitters and neuropeptides [1]. On the other hand, the glucocorticoid-mediated feedback mechanism, which takes place at pituitaric, hypothalamic and hippocampal levels, is the most important influence integrating the circadian activity of HPA axis and adapting the HPA response to stress [2-5].

Glucocorticoids (GCs) inhibit HPA axis through the activation of two distinct receptor types: type 1, or mineralocorticoid receptor (MR), and type 2, or glucocorticoid receptor (GR) [3, 4, 6-8]. Animal studies showed that GRs are distributed everywhere in the brain, mostly in hypothalamic neurons, as well as in corticotroph cells at the pituitary level [4,7], where they bind both natural and synthetic GCs [4]. On the contrary, MRs are mainly located in the limbic structures, in particular in the hippocampus [3,4,7,8], where they have lost aldosterone selectivity and bind GCs with affinity 10 fold higher than that displayed by GRs; thus, differently from GRs, MRs are mostly occupied at low GCs concentrations [4,7]. There is evidence both in animals and humans that hippocampal MRs mainly mediate the "proactive" feedback of GCs in the mantainance of basal HPA activity [4, 5, 9], through tonic inhibitory projections to the paraventricular nucleus [10-14]. On the other hand, the progressive occupancy of GRs following the increase of GCs concentrations is likely to mediate, in coordinated manner with MRs, the "reactive" feedback, aimed at controlling the HPA response to stress [4, 5, 9].

Aging as well as several physiopathological conditions, such as major depression, obesity, anorexia, have been shown associated with impaired HPA function, mainly connoted by functional hyperactivation due to impaired sensitivity to GCs feedback [4]. This hormonal abnormality has been suggested to be involved in the occurence of some clinical features that connotes either human aging or the above mentioned diseases [4]. To verify the activity of HPA axis in these conditions, in particular its response to GCs feedback, dexamenthasone-suppression test is usually used. Dexamethasone (DEX), is a synthetic GC with selectivity for GR that posseses an anti-inflammatory potency 30-40 times greater than that of endogenous GCs; however, it poorly penetrates blood-brain barrier (BBB) and preferentially activates pituitaric GRs [15-19]. For this reason, this compound should not conceptually represent the best tool to study the mechanisms involved in the feedback control of HPA axis that is mainly under CNS modulation. In fact, HPA impairment associated to aging, metabolic alterations or major depression mostly reflects abnormalities in the hippocampal sensitivity to GCs [4]. Conversely, endogenous GCs, such as corticosterone or cortisol, that easily cross the BBB, preferentially target the brain and exert their primary feedback on CNS areas, such as hippocampus and hypothalamus, by acting on both MR and GR [4,17]. Thus, it may be hypothesised that natural GCs could better evaluate the GC action on HPA function, particularly when central feedback is subject of investigation.

In this context, it has to be emphasized that the minimal effective dose of cortisol able to inhibit HPA activity in humans has never been definitely clarified. In previous human studies focusing on the GC feedback action, pharmachological cortisol doses have generally been used [20-23]. Moreover, to our knowledge, no human study has ever compared the effects of equipotent doses of natural and synthetic GCs on HPA function.

In this study we investigated the effect of various doses of either natural or synthetic GCs on HPA function in order to compare the effects of their equipotent doses in normal young volunteers.

Subjects and Methods

Drugs

Vials containing 100 mg hydrocortisone were purchased from Pharmacia & Upjohn S.p.A (Milan, Italy). Vials containing 4 mg dexamethasone were purchased from Biologici Italia Laboratories s.r.l. (Milan, Italy).

Study Protocol

Six normal subjects (all women; age, mean ± SEM: 25±2.1 yr; BMI: 23.0±1.2 kg/m^2) were studied. All subjects gave their informed consent to participate in the study which had been approved by an independent Ethical Committee. All subjects were studied in their follicular phase.

All subjects received the following treatments, in morning hours: 1) placebo (saline, 250 ml infused over 150 min from 08.00 to 10.30 h); 2) hydrocortisone at three different doses (HC, 15, 30 or 60 μg/kg/h, about 2.5, 5 and 10 mg, infused over 150 min from 08.00 to 10.30 h); 3) dexamethasone (DEX, 0.4, 0.8 or 1.6 μg/kg/h, about 0.07, 0.15 and 0.3 mg, infused over 150 min from 08.00 to 10.30 h). Blood samples were taken basally and then every 15 min up to +240 min. At each time point ACTH and cortisol levels were assayed. Treatment sessions were performed in random order at least 5 days apart, starting in the morning at 08.00 h after an overnight fast and 30 min after cannulation of a vein kept patent by slow infusion of isotonic saline.

Plasma ACTH levels (pg/ml; 0.22 pg/ml= 1 pmol/l) were measured in duplicate by immunoradiometric assay (Allegro HS-ACTH, IRMA, Nichols Institute Diagnostic, San Juan Capistrano, CA, USA). The sensitivity of the assay was 0.22 pg/ml. The inter-and intra-assay coefficients of variation ranged from 2.4 to 8.5 % and from 3.9 to 9.9 %, respectively.

Serum cortisol (μg/l; 2.7 μg/l= 1 nmol/l) was measured in duplicate by RIA (CORT-CTK125; DIA Sorin, Diasorin Diagnostics, Saluggia, Italy). The sensitivity of the assay was 11.0 μg/l. The inter-and intra-assay coefficient of variation ranged from 4.3 to 14.6 % and from 4.2 to 8.96 %, respectively.

All samples from an individual subject were analyzed together.

The results are expressed as mean ± SEM of absolute hormonal levels. The statistical analysis was carried out by using non-parametric ANOVA (Friedman test) and then Wilcoxon test when appropriate.

Results

During placebo, ACTH and cortisol levels showed progressive decrease (baseline vs nadir, mean±SEM: 17.6±1.6 vs 13.4±0.7 pg/ml and 157.6±25.6 vs 71.7±10.6 μg/l, $p<0.05$) (Tables 1 and 2, Figure 1 and 2). The dose of 15 μg/kg/h HC mantained constant cortisol levels but did not modify ACTH levels at any time. (Tables 1, Figure 1). Conversely, the doses 30 and 60 μg/kg/h HC induced dose-dependent cortisol increases (peaks, 30 μg/kg/h: 170.5±14.8 μg/l, $p<0.05$ vs the same placebo time point; 60 μg/kg/h: 203.2±26.6 μg/l, $p<0.05$ vs the same placebo time point) associated to dose-dependent ACTH decrease (nadir, 30 μg/kg/h: 8.1±0.9 pg/ml, $p<0.05$ vs the same placebo point; 60 μg/kg/h: 7.9±0.7 pg/ml, $p<0.05$ vs the same placebo point) (Table 1, Figure 1). The dose of 60 μg/kg/h HC more quickly decreased ACTH levels that persisted unchanged in the 90 minutes following the stop of HC infusion. Interestingly, after stopping 30 μg/kg/h HC, ACTH levels showed further decrease and became overlapping to those observed in the session where the highest HC dose had been administered. Despite no significant change in ACTH and cortisol during 15 μg/kg/h HC, after stopping the infusion, ACTH levels showed a further trend toward decrease. (Figure 1). DEX at doses of 0.4, 0.8 or 1.6 μg/kg/h did not significantly modify cortisol levels at any time. Neither 0.4 μg/kg/h nor 0.8 μg/kg/h DEX significantly modified ACTH levels at any time. The dose of 1.6 μg/kg/h DEX only induced an ACTH decrease significantly more pronounced than that during placebo (8.0±3.1 pg/ml, $p<0.05$ vs the same placebo time point). (Table 2, Figure 2).

Side Effects

No side effects were recorded after the administration of both HC or DEX at every dose.

Discussion

The results of the present study in young healthy subjects demonstrate that: 1) the HPA axis is sensitive to the inhibitory feedback action induced by very low HC doses, 30 μg/kg/h (5 mg) being the minimal effective dose able to inhibit ACTH levels; 2) equipotent doses of HC or DEX do not exert the same inhibitory effect on ACTH levels, being the minimal effective dose of DEX relatively higher than HC; 3) up to 1.6 μg/kg/h DEX dose is not able to modify the spontaneous cortisol secretion. In other words, taking into account the greater DEX potency at the GR level, doses of DEX relatively higher than HC are needed to inhibit HPA axis in humans. As anticipated, DEX, a synthetic glucocorticoid with a selective affinity for GR higher than HC, poorly penetrates BBB and therefore its negative feedback action is preferentially reflecting activation of GRs at the pituitary level [15-19]. Despite this evidence, the HPA feedback mechanisms are generally tested by using synthetic GCs, namely DEX generally at pharmacological doses [15]. This probably reduces the possibility to look for subtle changes in HPA sensitivity to feedback action, particularly in some conditions such as aging, major depression, visceral obesity, anorexia, that are connoted by functional hyperactivation of HPA axis probably associated to central hyposensitivity to GCs feedback [4]. This HPA hyperactivation would play a role in some clinical features connoting these conditions [4].

Table 1. Cortisol (μg/l; 2.7 μg/l= 1 nmol/l) and ACTH (pg/ml; 0.22 pg/ml= 1 pmol/l) levels (baseline, peaks and nadir, mean±SEM) after placebo or hydrocortisone (HC) infusion at different doses (15, 30 or 60 μg/kg/h) in normal subjects

	cortisol (μg/l)			ACTH (pg/ml)		
	baseline	peaks	nadir	baseline	peaks	nadir
Placebo	157.6±25.6	-	71.7±10.6	17.6±1.6	-	13.4±0.7
HC 15 μg/kg/h	146.1±14.3	-	81.7±10.8	21.6±2.8	-	11.2±2.2
HC 30 μg/kg/h	149.8±15.2	170.5±14.8 *	105.2±8.3	22.0±2.0	-	8.1±0.9 *
HC 60 μg/kg/h	143.4±15.1	203.2±26.6 *	134.4±15.6	18.5±2.2	-	7.9±0.7 *

*P<0.05 vs the same placebo time point.

Table 2. Cortisol (μg/l; 2.7 μg/l= 1 nmol/l) and ACTH (pg/ml; 0.22 pg/ml= 1 pmol/l) levels (baseline, peaks and nadir, mean±SEM) after placebo or dexamethasone (DEX) infusion at different doses (0.4, 0.8 or 1.6 μg/kg/h) in normal subjects

		cortisol (μg/l)			ACTH (pg/ml)	
	baseline	peaks	nadir	baseline	peaks	nadir
placebo	157.6±25.6	-	71.7±10.6	17.6±1.6	-	13.4±0.7
DEX 0.4 μg/kg/h	191.6±37.1	-	64.6±10.9	20.2±1.8	-	12.3±1.8
DEX 0.8 μg/kg/h	167.6±18.1	-	57.4±3.1	19.5±3.1	-	11.2±2.6
DEX 1.6 μg/kg/h	148.8±22.1	-	42.9±7.5	25.0±5.7	-	8.0±3.1 *

*$P<0.05$ vs the same placebo time point.

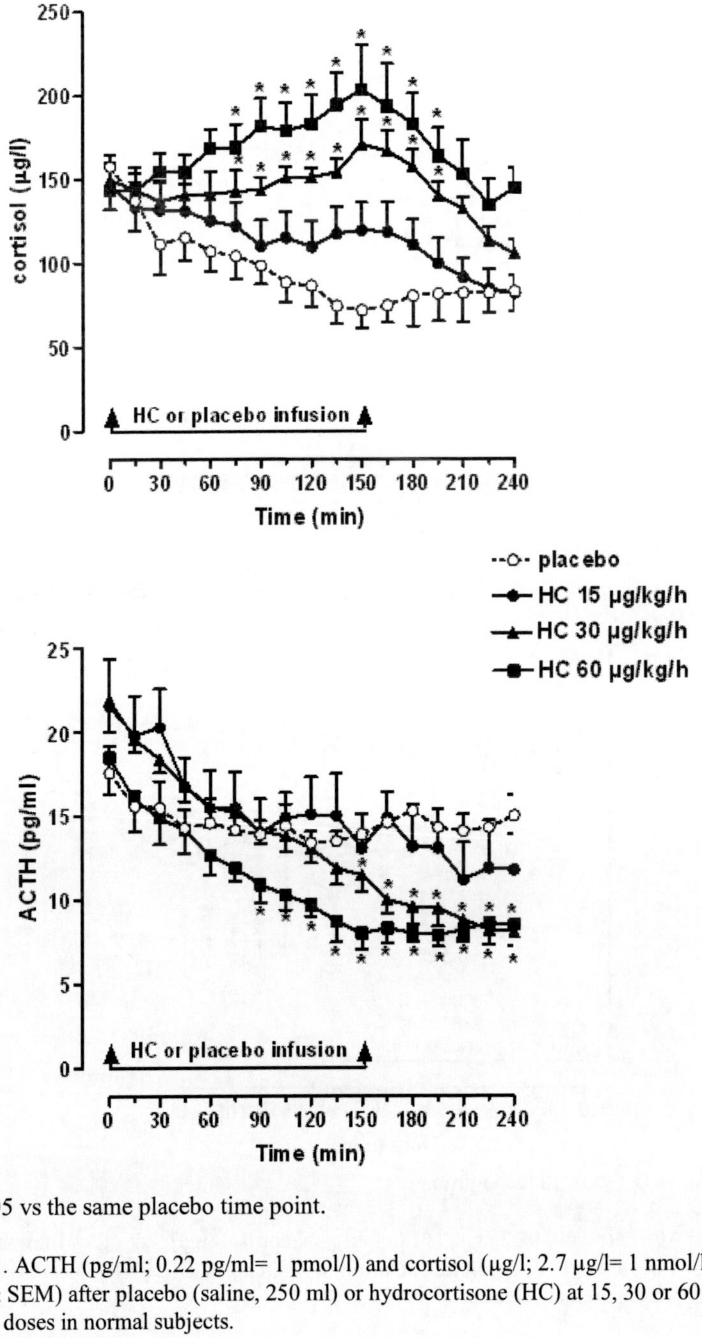

* P<0.05 vs the same placebo time point.

Figure 1. ACTH (pg/ml; 0.22 pg/ml= 1 pmol/l) and cortisol (µg/l; 2.7 µg/l= 1 nmol/l) levels (mean ± SEM) after placebo (saline, 250 ml) or hydrocortisone (HC) at 15, 30 or 60 µg/kg/h doses in normal subjects.

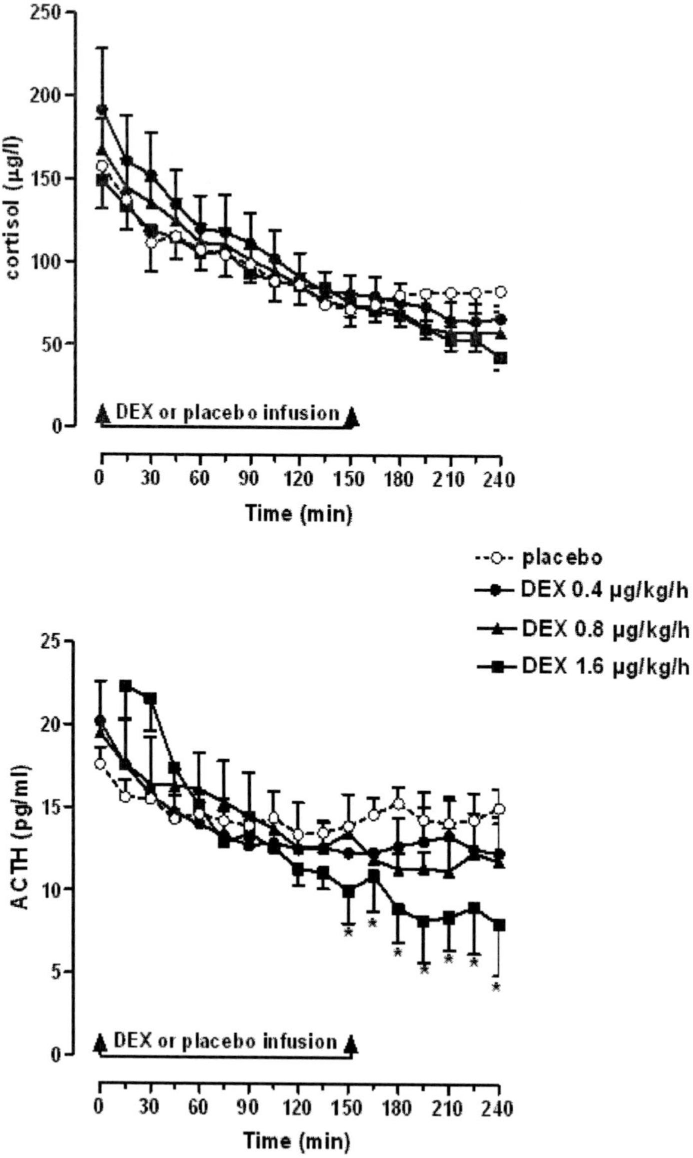

* P<0.05 vs the same placebo time point.

Figure 2. ACTH (pg/ml; 0.22 pg/ml= 1 pmol/l) and cortisol (µg/l; 2.7 µg/l= 1 nmol/l) levels (mean ± SEM) after placebo (saline, 250 ml) or dexamethasone (DEX) at 0.4, 0.8 or 1.6 µg/kg/h doses in normal subjects.

Herein we show that, taking into account the potency at the GR level, doses of DEX relatively higher than HC are needed to inhibit ACTH secretion in humans. In fact, the minimal effective doses of DEX and HC able to inhibit ACTH levels were 1.6 μg/kg/h (0.3 mg as total dose) and 30 μg/kg/h (5 mg as total dose), respectively. It has to be emphasized that even this highest DEX dose did not affect all the spontaneous cortisol secretion recorded after placebo administration. Considering that the affinity of DEX at the GR level is 30-40 times higher than that of HC, we expect a significantly minimal effective dose of DEX able to exert clear negative feedback action on HPA axis, i.e. ACTH and cortisol secretion.

On the other hand, evidence that a very low HC dose, i.e. approximately 5 mg, is already able to exert an inhibitory effect on ACTH secretion indicates that the HPA response is sensitive to cortisol concentrations clearly lower than those generally used in the previous studies [20-23]. As anticipated this HC dose is relatively lower than that of DEX needed but exerts clear inhibitory effect on ACTH secretion.

As expected, increasing doses of HC, augmented in a dose-dependent way circulating cortisol levels and decreased ACTH levels. The highest HC dose was able to decrease more quickly ACTH levels that persisted unchanged in the 90 minutes after stopping HC infusion. Interestingly, after stopping the intermediate HC dose, ACTH levels showed further decrease and became overlapping to those observed in the session where the highest HC dose had been administered. Again, despite no significant changes in ACTH and cortisol levels were recorded during the lowest HC dose, ACTH levels tended to decrease after stopping the infusion.

More prolonged observation of ACTH secretion after infusion's withdrawal could have allowed to see whether the lowest HC dose, that did not increase cortisol levels above baseline, could have some delayed negative feedback effect on corticotroph secretion.

In all, our present findings indicate that HPA axis display preferential sensitivity to the negative feedback action of cortisol. This would reflect the preferential central action of cortisol that crosses the BBB and can well act on hypothalamic GR as well as on both GR and MR at the hyppocampal level. Evidence that MRs are the first receptors occupied by low GC level fit well with our hypothesis.

Our findings also imply that DEX is likely to less appropriately explore the central mechanisms governing the GCs feedback control of HPA axis. This hypothesis is relevant considering that the investigation of subtle alterations in HPA sensitivity to feedback action need a more sensitive approach that could be well represented by administering submaximal doses of natural GCs. This consideration particulalrly applies to the clinical conditions considered above.

Conclusion

In conclusion, the results of the present study show that doses of dexamethasone relatively higher than hydrocortisone are needed to inhibit ACTH secretion in humans. These findings are likely to reflect different sites where natural and synthetic GCs exert their feedback action, i.e. mainly the CNS for hydrocortisone and the pituitary for dexamethasone.

Acknowledgments

This study was supported by a grant from University of Turin, and Foundation for the Study of Endocrine and Metabolic Diseases.

References

[1] Orth, DN.Corticotropin-releasing hormone in humans.*Endocrine Reviews*1992 13,164-191.

[2] Gaillard, RC; Al Damluji, S. Stress and the pituitary-adrenal axis.*Baillieres Clinical Endocrinology and Metabolism* 1987 1,319-354.

[3] Jacobson, L;Sapolsky, R.The role of the hippocampus in feedback regulation of the hypothalamic- pituitary adrenocortical axis.*Endocrine Reviews*1991 12,118-134.

[4] de Kloet, ER;Vreugdenhil, E;Oitzl, MS;Joels, M. Brain corticosteroid receptor balance in health and disease. *Endocrine Reviews* 1998 19,269-301.

[5] Sapolsky, R; Romero, ML;Munck, AU. How do glucocorticoids influence stress responses? Integrating permissive, suppressive, stimulatory and preparative actions.*Endocrine Reviews* 2000 21, 55-89.

[6] Ratka, A;Sutanto, W;Bloemers, M; de Kloet, ER.On the role of brain mineralocorticoid (type I) and glucocorticoid (type II) receptors in neuroendocrine regulation.*Neuroendocrinology*198950,117-123.

[7] Funder, JW. Glucocorticoid and mineralocorticoid receptors: biology and clinical relevance. *Annual Review of Medicine* 1997 48,231-240.

[8] Berardelli, R; Karamouzis, I; D'Angelo, V; Zichi, C; Fussotto, B; Giordano, R; Ghigo, E; Arvat, E. Role of the mineralcorticoid receptors on HPA axis in humans.*Endocrine* 2013 43, 51-58.

[9] Won, JG; Jap, TS; Chang, SC;Ching, KN; Chiang, BN. Evidence for a delayed, integral, and proportional phase of glucocorticoid feedback on ACTH secretion in normal human volunteers. *Metabolism* 1986 35,254-259.

[10] Swanson, LW;Sawchenko, PE; Lind, RW; Rho, JH. The CRH motoneuron: differential peptide regulation in neurons with possible synaptic, paracrine, and endocrine outputs. *Annals of the New York Academic of Sciences* 1987 512,12-23.

[11] Swanson, LW. Biochemical switching in hypothalamic circuits mediating responses to stress.*Progress in Brain Research* 199187,181-200.

[12] Herman, JP; Prewitt, CM;Cullinan, WE.Neuronal circuit regulation of the hypothalamo-pituitary-adrenocortical stress axis.*Critical Reviews in Neurobiology* 199610,371-394.

[13] Erkut, ZA; Pool, C;Swaab, DF. Glucocorticoids suppress corticotropin-releasing hormone and vasopressin expression in human hypothalamic neurons. *Journal of Clinical Endocrinology and Metabolism* 1998 83,2066-2073.

[14] Herman, JP; Watson, SJ; Spencer, RL.Defense of adrenocorticosteroid receptor expression in rat hippocampus: effects of stress and strain. *Endocrinology* 1999 140,3981-3991.

[15] Miller, AH; Spencer, RL;Pulera, M; Kang, S; McEwen, BS; Stein M. Adrenal steroid receptor activation in rat brain and pituitary following dexamethasone: implication for the dexamethasone suppression test. *Biological Psychiatry* 1992 32, 850-869.

[16] Meijer, OC; de Lange, EC;Breimer, DD; de Boer, AG;Workel, JO; de Kloet, ER. Penetration of dexamethasone into brain glucocorticoid targets is enhanced in mdr1A P-glycoprotein knockout mice. *Endocrinology* 1998 139, 1789-1793.

[17] Kovacs, KJ;Makara, GB.Corticosterone and dexamethasone act at different brain sites to inhibit adrenalectomy-induced adrenocorticotropinhypersecretion. *Brain Research*1988 474, 205-210.

[18] Cole, MA; Kim, PJ;Kalman, BA; Spencer RL. Dexamethasone suppression of corticosteroid secretion: evaluation of the site of action

by receptor measures and functional studies. *Psychoneuroendocrinology* 2000 25, 151-167.

[19] Feldman, S;Weidenfeld, J.Further evidence for the central effect of dexamethasone at the hypothalamic level in the negative feedback mechanism.*Brain Research*2002 958, 291-296.

[20] Wilkinson, CW;Peskind, ER;Raskinf, MA.Decreased hypothalamic-pituitary-adrenal axis sensitivity to cortisol feedback inhibition in human aging.*Neuroendocrinology* 1997 65, 79-90.

[21] Posener, JA;Schildkraut, JJ; Williams, GH;Schatzberg, AF. Cortisol feedback effects on plasma corticotropin levels in healthy subjects. *Psychoneuroendocrinology* 1997 22,169-176 .

[22] Posener, JA;Schildkraut, JJ; Williams, GH;Schatzberg, AF. Late feedback effects of hypothalamic-pituitary-adrenal axis hormones in healthy subjects. *Psychoneuroendocrinology* 1998 23, 371-383.

[23] Boscaro, M;Paoletta, A;Scarpa, E;Barzon, L;Fusaro, P;Fallo, F;Sonino, N. Age-related changes in glucocorticoid fast feedback inhibition of adrenocorticotropin in man. *Journal of Clinical Endocrinology and Metabolism* 1998 83,1380-1383.

In: Dexamethasone
Editors: A. Sauvage and M. Levy
ISBN: 978-1-62808-405-4

Chapter VII

Effect of Dexamethasone on Parathyroid Hormone-related Protein Expression by Oral Cancer Cells

Masatoshi Abe
Division of Chemistry, Department of Biomaterials Science,
Ohu University School of Dentistry, Tomita-machi, Koriyama, Japan

Abstract

Parathyroid hormone-related protein (PTHrP) is known to act as a major causative factor for humoral hypercalcemia of malignancy (HHM). Production of PTHrP is up-regulated in certain malignancies and elevated PTHrP expression has been correlated with advanced disease and a poor prognosis. Therefore, down-regulation of PTHrP production in cancer cells is important to provide an approach for prevention of HHM. But there is little effective treatment for controlling the increased production of PTHrP in cancer cells. Glucocorticoids (including dexamethasone) exhibit diverse biological activities, such as anti-inflammatory and immunosuppressive effects on various cells and tissues. There is also considerable interest in application of glucocorticoids to cancer treatment. In the latest research using HSC-3, a human oral squamous carcinoma cell line, it was demonstrated that dexamethasone suppresses PTHrP mRNA expression and PTHrP production in a dose-dependent manner. Furthermore, dexamethasone was shown to act through binding to functional glucocorticoid receptors and down-regulate PTHrP gene expression via a transcriptional mechanism in HSC-3 cells. Application of dexamethasone may become a new strategy for preventing PTHrP-induced HHM .

Introduction

Parathyroid hormone-related protein (PTHrP) [1-5] was first identified as a major causative factor for humoral hypercalcemia of malignancy (HHM). PTHrP acts on the bones and kidneys, and its *in vivo* biological effects include an increase of bone resorption and phosphaturia, as well as elevated urinary excretion of cAMP, resembling the actions of parathyroid hormone [6,7]. PTHrP has been shown to be expressed by a range of tumor cell lines and solid tumors. PTHrP produced by neoplastic cells stimulates osteoclastic bone resorption and renal reabsorption of calcium by binding to PTH/PTHrP receptors in the bones and kidneys, thus leading to hypercalcemia [8]. In hypercalcemic patients with cancer, elevated PTHrP expression has been correlated with advanced disease and a poor prognosis [9,10]. However, PTHrP is also expressed in many normal tissues, including normal human keratinocytes, mammary glands, and aortic smooth muscle cells. In addition to its endocrine actions associated with the development of HHM, PTHrP is known to act as an autocrine/paracrine factor that regulates differentiation and proliferation in normal tissues [11-13].

The molecular mechanism by which PTHrP production is up-regulated in certain malignancies and its role in cellular transformation remain unknown. In addition, there is little effective treatment for controlling the increased production of PTHrP in cancer cells.

A number of regulators of PTHrP expression have been defined [14], and the majority of them have been found to enhance PTHrP mRNA and protein levels. Growth factors (EGF, TGF-β, etc.), cAMP, calcium, cycloheximide, and the *tax* gene product are some of the up-regulators, while down-regulators of PTHrP expression include certain ligands for nuclear receptors [15] such as 1,25-dihydroxyvitamin D_3 ($1,25(OH)_2D_3$), dexamethasone, and testosterone. Down-regulation of PTHrP production in cancer cells is important to provide an approach for prevention of HHM.

Glucocorticoids (including dexamethasone) exhibit diverse biological activities, such as anti-inflammatory and immunosuppressive effects on various cells and tissues. There is also considerable interest in application of glucocorticoids to cancer treatment. In the latest research, effect of dexamethasone on PTHrP mRNA expression and PTHrP production was examined using HSC-3 [16], a human oral squamous carcinoma cell line.

Effect of Dexamethasone on PTHrP Expression

In certain malignancies, PTHrP gene expression is up-regulated, leading to the development of HHM [8]. The molecular mechanism by which PTHrP gene expression is activated in some malignant cells remains to be clarified, and there are few effective approaches for controlling increased tumor cell production of PTHrP.

HSC-3 cells expressed PTHrP mRNA and secreted PTHrP into conditioned medium under basal conditions [17]. A prominent transcript for PTHrP was expressed at 1.5 kb in HSC-3 cells. The effect of dexamethasone on PTHrP mRNA expression by HSC-3 cells was examined with Northern blot analysis. As shown in Figure 1(A) and Figure 1(B), dexamethasone down-regulated PTHrP mRNA expression in a concentration-dependent manner [18]. Marked suppression was observed at concentrations of 10^{-7} M and 10^{-6} M, with the PTHrP mRNA level falling to less than 30% of that in vehicle-treated control cells [18]. In order to determine whether dexamethasone not only decreased PTHrP mRNA expression but also PTHrP secretion by HSC-3 cells, the PTHrP concentration in the conditioned medium was measured by IRMA using two antibodies with epitopes of human PTHrP (1-34) and PTHrP (50-83). As shown in Figure 1(C), dexamethasone decreased PTHrP secretion in a concentration-dependent manner [18]. At 10^{-6} M, PTHrP secretion was reduced by 37% relative to that of control cells [18]. The time course of the effect of dexamethasone on PTHrP mRNA expression was also determined by using HSC-3 cells treated with 10^{-7} M dexamethasone (data not shown). A significant decrease in PTHrP mRNA abundance was observed as early as 6 h after the initiation of dexamethasone treatment, and this suppressive effect was stronger at 24 h [18]. These findings indicate that dexamethasone is effective for suppressing PTHrP expression in HSC-3 cells.

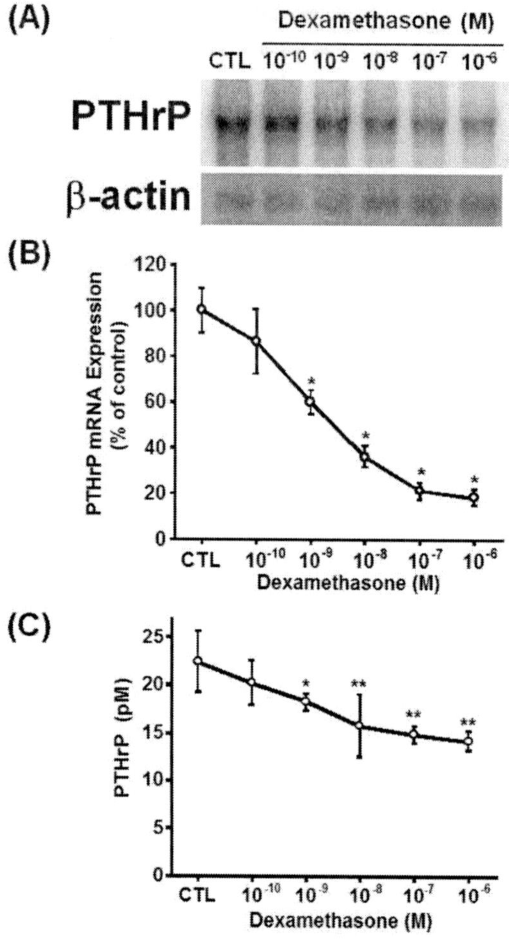

Figure 1. Concentration-response effect of dexamethasone on PTHrP mRNA expression and PTHrP secretion by HSC-3 cells. HSC-3 cells were incubated with various concentrations of dexamethasone in serum-free DMEM for 24 h. (A) Total RNA (20 μg) was subjected to Northern blot analysis for PTHrP and β-actin mRNAs. (B) PTHrP mRNA was quantified by densitometric analysis of the Northern blots, and its level was normalized for that of β-actin mRNA. Data are expressed as the mean±S.D. of triplicate determinations. *: $p<0.01$ compared with vehicle control (CTL). (C) The immunoreactive PTHrP concentration in the medium was measured by IRMA. Data are expressed as the mean±S.D. of triplicate determinations. *: $p<0.05$ and **: $p<0.01$ compared with the vehicle control (CTL).

Transcriptional regulation of the human PTHrP gene is achieved by three distinct promoters, which have been designated as P1, P2, and P3 [20-22].

Several studies have shown that usage of the downstream promoter (P2/P3) is common in many cancers [23-25]. Therefore, a luciferase reporter plasmid containing the downstream promoter (P2/P3) region of the human PTHrP gene was constructed and was transiently transfected into HSC-3 cells. Transcriptional activity was evaluated by the luciferase reporter assay. As shown in Figure 3, the transcriptional activity of the PTHrP promoter was reduced by 33% in dexamethasone-treated cells [18]. This result suggested that dexamethasone down-regulates PTHrP gene expression via a transcriptional mechanism in HSC-3 cells.

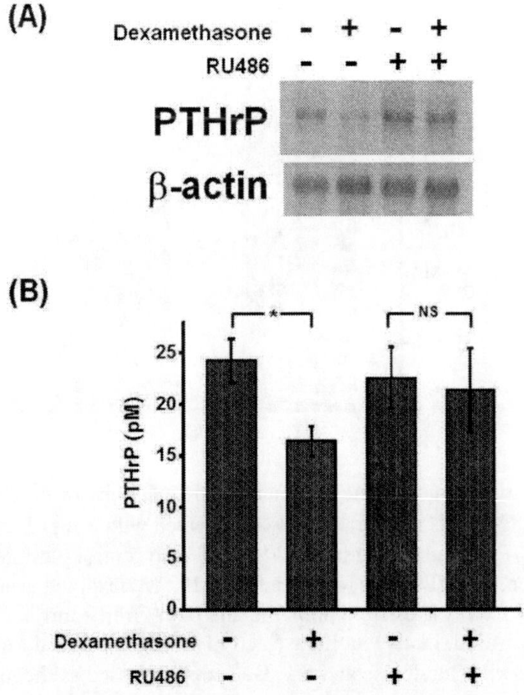

Figure 2. Effect of RU486 on dexamethasone-mediated suppression of PTHrP mRNA expression and PTHrP secretion by HSC-3 cells. HSC-3 cells were pretreated with 10^{-6} M RU486 in serum-free DMEM for 1 h, and then were incubated with the vehicle or 10^{-7} M dexamethasone in the presence of RU486 for 24 h. Cells incubated without RU486 were grown with the vehicle. (A) Total RNA (20 μg) was subjected to Northern blot analysis for PTHrP and β-actin mRNAs. (B) The immunoreactive PTHrP concentration in the culture medium was measured by IRMA. Data are expressed as the mean±S.D. of triplicate determinations. *: p<0.01 compared with the vehicle control (CTL). NS : no significant difference.

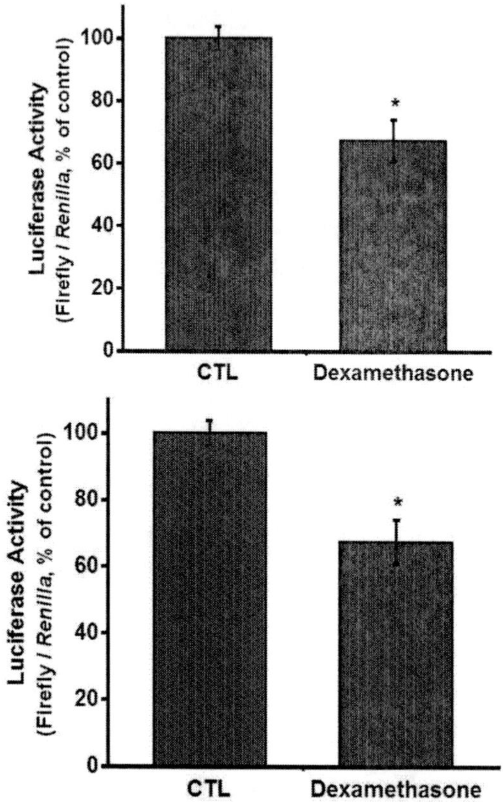

Figure 3. Effect of dexamethasone on transcriptional activity of the PTHrP promoter in HSC-3 cells. HSC-3 cells were transiently transfected with 2 μg of luciferase reporter plasmid (PTHrP-Luc) and 0.1 μg of *Renilla* luciferase control plasmid (pRL-TK). After transfection, the cells were incubated with 10^{-7} M dexamethasone in serum-free DMEM for 48 h. Cell lysates were prepared and both Firefly and *Renilla* luciferase activity were measured. Firefly luciferase activity was normalized for the corresponding *Renilla* luciferase activity. Data are expressed as the mean±S.D. of quadruplicate determinations. *: $p<0.01$ compared with the vehicle control (CTL).

Mechanism of Dexamethasone Action

Generally, glucocorticoids exert their biological effects through binding glucocorticoid receptors (GRs) which are a class of nuclear receptors that act as ligand-dependent transcription factors [19]. To explore the role of the GR in the regulation of PTHrP expression by dexamethasone, the GR antagonist

RU486 was employed. HSC-3 cells were pretreated with a 10-fold molar excess of RU486 prior to the addition of dexamethasone. As shown in Figure 2(A), dexamethasone-induced suppression of PTHrP mRNA expression was abolished in the presence of RU486 [18]. This finding indicates that the suppressive effect of dexamethasone arises through its binding to functional GRs. In agreement with the above-mentioned result, the dexamethasone-induced decrease in PTHrP secretion was also abolished in the presence of RU486 (Figure 2(B)) [18].

Glucocorticoids (including dexamethasone) exert their anti-inflammatory and anti-proliferative effects principally by inhibiting the expression of various cytokines and adhesion molecules. Glucocorticoids bind to the GR, and then this GR complex undergoes translocation to the nucleus. A ligand-activated homodimer of GR binds to the glucocorticoid-response element (GRE) in the promoter sequence upstream of each target gene and thus exerts transcriptional regulation [19]. Depending on the target gene, binding of the GR to the GRE may either enhance or repress transcriptional activity. In contrast to the GRE that mediates stimulation of gene transcription, a negative GRE (nGRE) [26] inhibits the gene expression promoted by glucocorticoids. In addition to transcriptional regulation mediated by GR-GRE interaction, glucocorticoids can repress gene transcription by antagonizing the activity and/or function of various transcription factors. For example, ligand-activated GR represses the nuclear translocation and/or function of the transcription factors AP-1 [27,28], NF-κB [29,30], and NF-AT [31,32].

Among the factors that down-regulate PTHrP gene expression, the action of $1,25(OH)_2D_3$ has been studied extensively. Three negative vitamin D-response elements (nVDREs) have been identified in the rat PTHrP promoter [33,34], while one nVDRE has been identified in the human PTHrP promoter [35]. The precise mechanism by which dexamethasone regulates PTHrP gene expression remains unclear. There is no evidence that ligand-activated GR directly interacts with a specific DNA element in the PTHrP promoter, so an nGRE has not yet been identified in this promoter. It has been shown that dexamethasone suppresses the expression of certain genes without GR-nGRE interaction. Dexamethasone-induced suppression of collagenase-1 gene expression is mediated by the interaction of activated GR with AP-1 [28]. Activated GR also suppresses interleukin-6 gene expression by directly interfering with the function of NF-κB [29]. Through protein-protein interaction, dexamethasone-activated GR might possibly antagonize a transcription factor that constitutively binds to the PTHrP promoter and elicits transcriptional activity. But the possibility that GRE might be present at the site very near the binding site of a constitutive transcription factor can not be excluded.

PTHrP production is known to be up-regulated in certain malignancies, and PTHrP gene expression is stimulated by several growth factors in many types of cells [14]. Ets-1 binding site [36] is present in the sequence of P3 promoter that is used most frequently among the three promoters of PTHrP in several cancer cells [23-25], and Ets-1 is crucial for basal transcriptional activity of the promoter. Ets-1 functions as a downstream target of Ras/MAP kinase pathway [37] that is activated by certain growth factors including EGF, a potent stimulator of PTHrP expression. Lindemann et al. [38] have reported that an interaction between Smad3 and Ets-1 is involved in the TGF-β-stimulated PTHrP gene expression in breast cancer cells. With regard to the action of dexamethasone on PTHrP expression in HSC-3 cells, one possibility is that the function of Ets-1 might be inhibited by activated GR leading to down-regulation of transcriptional activity of PTHrP P3 promoter.

Conclusion

Dexamethasone was found to suppress PTHrP mRNA expression and PTHrP production by HSC-3 cells in a dose-dependent manner. Furthermore, dexamethasone was shown to act through binding to functional glucocorticoid receptors and down-regulate PTHrP gene expression via a transcriptional mechanism in HSC-3 cells. Application of dexamethasone may become a new strategy for preventing PTHrP-induced HHM .

References

[1] Moseley, J. M., Kubota, M., Diefenbach-Jagger, H., Wettenhall, R. E. H., Kemp, B. E., Suva, L. J., Rodda, C. P., Ebeling, P. R., Hudson, P. J., Zajac, J. D. & Martin, T. J. (1987). Parathyroid hormone-related protein purified from a human lung cancer cell line. *Proc. Natl. Acad. Sci. USA, 84*, 5048-5052.

[2] Suva, L. J., Winslow, G. A., Wettenhall, R. E. H., Hammonds, R. G., Moseley, J. M., Diefenbach-Jagger, H., Rodda, C. P., Kemp, B. E., Rodriguez, H., Chen, E. Y., Hudson, P. J., Martin, T. J. & Wood, W. I.

(1987). A parathyroid hormone-related protein implicated in malignant hypercalcemia : cloning and expression. *Science, 237*, 893-896.

[3] Mangin, M., Webb, A. C., Dreyer, B. E., Posillico, J. T., Ikeda, K., Weir, W. C., Stewart, A. F., Bander, N. H., Milstone, L., Barton, D. E., Francke, U. & Broadus, A. E. (1988). Identification of a cDNA encoding a parathyroid hormone-like peptide from a human tumor associated with humoral hypercalcemia of malignancy. *Proc. Natl. Acad. Sci. USA*, *85*, 597-601.

[4] Thiede, M. A., Strewler, G. J., Nissenson, R. A., Rosenblatt, M. & Rodan, G. A. (1988). Human renal carcinoma expresses two messages encoding a parathyroid hormone-like peptide : evidence for the alternative splicing of a single copy gene. *Proc. Natl. Acad. Sci. USA, 85*, 4605-4609.

[5] Yasuda, T., Banville, D., Rabbani, S. A., Hendy, G. N. & Goltzman D. (1989). Rat parathyroid hormone-like peptide : comparison with the human homologue and expression in malignant and normal tissue. *Mol. Endocrinol., 3*, 518-525.

[6] Horiuchi, N., Caulfield, M. P., Fisher, J. E., Goldman, M. E., McKee, R. L., Reagan, J. E., Levy, J. J., Nutt, R. F., Rodan, S. B., Schofield, T. L., Clements, T. L. & Rosenblatt, M. (1987). Similarity of synthetic peptide from human tumor to parathyroid hormone *in vivo* and *in vitro*. *Science, 238*, 1566-1568.

[7] Kemp, B. E., Moseley, J. M., Rodda, C. P., Ebeling, P. R., Wettenhall, R. E. H., Stapleton, D., Diefenbach-Jagger, H., Ure, F., Michelangeli, V. P., Simmons, H. A., Raisz, L. G. & Nartin, T. J. (1987). Parathyroid hormone-related protein of malignancy : active synthetic fragments. *Science, 238*, 1568-1570.

[8] Rosol, T. J. & Capen, C. C. (1992). Mechanisms of cancer-induced hypercalcemia. *Lab. Invest., 67*, 680-702.

[9] Pecherstorfer, M., Schilling, T., Blind, E., Zimmer-Roth, I., Baumgartner, G., Ziegler, R. & Raue, F. (1994). Parathyroid hormone-related protein and life expectancy in hypercalcemic cancer patients. *J. Clin. Endocrinol. Metab., 78*, 1268-1270.

[10] Yoshida, A., Nakamura, Y., Shimizu, A., Harada, M., Kameda, Y., Nagano, A., Inaba, M. & Asaga, T. (2000). Significance of the Parathyroid hormone-related protein expression in breast carcinoma. *Breast Cancer, 7*, 215-220.

[11] Philbrick, W. M., Wysolmerski, J. J., Galbraith, S., Holt, E., Orloff, J. J., Yang, K. H., Vasavada, R. C., Weir, E. C., Broadus, A. E. & Stewart, A.

F. (1996). Defining the role of parathyroid hormone-related protein in normal physiology. *Physiol. Rev., 76*, 127-173.

[12] Strewler, G. J. (2000). The physiology of parathyroid hormone-related protein. *N. Engl. J. Med., 342*, 177-185.

[13] Moseley, J. M. & Gillespie, M. T. (1995). Parathyroid hormone-related protein. *Crit. Rev. Clin. Lab. Sci., 32*, 299-343.

[14] Gillespie, M. T. & Martin, T. J. (1994). The parathyroid hormone-related protein gene and its expression. *Mol. Cell. Endocrinol., 100*, 143-147.

[15] Evans, R. M. (1988). The steroid and thyroid hormone receptor superfamily. *Science, 240*, 889-895.

[16] Kamata, N., Chida, K., Rikimaru, K., Horikoshi, M., Enomoto, S. & Kuroki, T. (1986). Growth-inhibitory effects of epidermal growth factor and overexpression of its receptors on human squamous cell carcinomas in culture. *Cancer Res., 46*, 1648-1653.

[17] Abe, M., Akeno, N., Ohida, S. & Horiuchi, N. (1998). Inhibitory effects of 1,25-dihydroxyvitamin D_3 and 9-*cis*-retinoic acid on parathyroid hormone-related protein expression by oral cancer cells (HSC-3). *J. Endocrinol., 156*, 349-357.

[18] Abe, M., & Horiuchi, N. (2010). Dexamethasone suppresses parathyroid hormone-related protein expression by human oral squamous carcinoma cells (HSC-3). *J. Oral Biosci., 52*, 51-59.

[19] Gower, W. R. Jr. (1993). Mechanism of glucocorticoid action. *J. Fla. Med. Assoc., 80*, 697-700.

[20] Mangin, M., Ikeda, M., Dreyer, B. E. & Broadus, A. E. (1990). Identification of an up-stream promoter of the human parathyroid hormone-related peptide gene. *Mol. Endocrinol., 4*, 851-858.

[21] Vasavada, R. C., Wysolmerski, J. J., Broadus, A. E. & Philbrick, W. M. (1993). Identification and characterization of a GC-rich promoter of the human parathyroid hormone-related peptide gene. *Mol. Endocrinol., 7*, 273-282.

[22] Suva, L. J., Mather, K. A., Gillespie, M. T., Webb, G. C., Ng, K. W., Winslow, G. A., Wood, W. I., Martin, T. J. & Hudson, P. J. (1989). Structure of the 5' flanking region of the gene encoding human parathyroid hormone-related protein (PTHrP). *Gene, 77*, 95-105.

[23] Bouizar, Z., Spyratos, F. & De Vernejoul, M. C. (1999). The parathyroid hormone-related protein (PTHrP) gene: use of downstream TATA promoter and PTHrP 1-139 coding pathways in primary breast cancers

vary with the occurrence of bone metastasis. *J. Bone Miner. Res., 14*, 406-414.

[24] Southby, J., Murphy, L. M., Martin, T. J. & Gillespie, M. T. (1996). Cell-specific and regulator-induced promoter usage and messenger ribonucleic acid splicing for parathyroid hormone-related protein. *Endocrinology, 137*, 1349-1357.

[25] Richard, V., Luchin, A., Brena, R. M., Plass, C. & Rosol, T. J. (2003). Quantitative evaluation of alternative promoter usage and 3' splice variants for parathyroid hormone-related protein by real-time reverse transcription-PCR. *Clin. Chem., 49*, 1398-1402.

[26] Dostert, A. & Heinzel, T. (2004). Negative glucocorticoid receptor response elements and their role in glucocorticoid action. *Curr. Pharm. Des., 10*, 2807-2816.

[27] Jonat, C., Rahmsdorf, H. J., Park, K. K., Cato, A. C., Gebel, S., Ponta, H. & Herrlich, P. (1990). Antitumor promotion and antiinflammation : down-modulation of AP-1 (Fos/Jun) activity by glucocorticoid hormone. *Cell, 62*, 1189-1204.

[28] Yang-Yen, H. F., Chambard, J. C., Sun, Y. L., Smeal, T., Schmidt, T. J., Drouin, J. & Karin, M. (1990). Transcriptional interference between c-Jun and the glucocorticoid receptor: mutual inhibition of DNA binding due to direct protein-protein interaction. *Cell, 62*, 1205-1215.

[29] De Bosscher, K., Schmitz, M. L., Vanden Berghe, W., Plaisance, S., Fiers, W. & Haegeman, G. (1997). Glucocorticoid-mediated repression of nuclear factor-kappaB-dependent transcription involves direct interference with transactivation. *Proc. Natl. Acad. Sci. USA, 94*, 13504-13509.

[30] Heck, S., Bender, K., Kullmann, M., Gottlicher, M., Herrlich, P. & Cato, A. C. (1997). I kappaB alpha-independent downregulation of NF-kappaB activity by glucocorticoid receptor. *EMBO J., 16*, 4698-4707.

[31] Paliogianni, F., Raptis, A., Ahuja, S. S., Najjar, S. M. & Boumpas, D. T. (1993). Negative transcriptional regulation of interleukin 2 (IL-2) gene by glucocorticoids through interference with nuclear transcription factors AP-1 and NF-AT. *J. Clin. Invest., 91*, 1481-1489.

[32] Chen, R., Burke, T. F., Cumberland, J. E., Brummet, M., Beck, L. A., Casolaro, V. & Georas, S. N. (2000). Glucocorticoids inhibit calcium- and calcineurin-dependent activation of the human IL-4 promoter. *J. Immunol., 164*, 825-832.

[33] Kremer, R., Sebag, M., Champigny, C., Meerovitch, K., Hendy, G. N., White, J. & Goltzman, D. (1996). Identification and characterization of

1,25-dihydroxyvitamin D_3-responsive repressor sequences in the rat parathyroid hormone-related peptide gene. *J. Biol. Chem., 271*, 16310-16316.

[34] Falzon, M. (1996). DNA sequences in the rat parathyroid hormone-related peptide gene responsible for 1,25-dihydroxyvitamin D_3-mediated transcriptional repression. *Mol. Endocrinol., 10*, 672-681.

[35] Nishishita, T., Okazaki, T., Ishikawa, T., Igarashi, T., Hata, K., Ogata, E. & Fujita, T. (1998). A negative vitamin D response DNA element in the human parathyroid hormone-related peptide gene binds to vitamin D receptor along with Ku antigen to mediate negative gene regulation by vitamin D. *J. Biol. Chem., 273*, 10901-10907.

[36] Richard, V., Rosol, T. J. & Foley, J. (2005). PTHrP gene expression in cancer : do all paths lead to Ets? *Crit. Rev. Eukaryot Gene Expr., 15*, 115-132.

[37] Wasylyk, C., Bradford, A. P., Gutierrez-Hartmann, A. & Wasylyk, B. (1997). Conserved mechanisms of Ras regulation of evolutionary related transcription factors, Ets1 and Pointed P2. *Oncogene, 14*, 899-913.

[38] Lindemann, R. K., Ballschmieter, P., Nordheim, A. & Dittmer, J. (2001). Transforming growth factor β regulates parathyroid hormone-related protein expression in MDA-MB-231 breast cancer cells through a novel Smad/Ets synergism. *J. Biol. Chem., 276*, 46661-46670.

In: Dexamethasone
Editors: A. Sauvage and M. Levy
ISBN: 978-1-62808-405-4

Chapter VIII

The Effects of Dexamethasone on the Proliferation and Differentiation of the Osteoblasts

Jun-Beom Park*

Department of Periodontics,
Seoul St Mary's Hospital, College of Medicine,
Catholic University of Korea, Seoul, Korea

Abstract

Dexamethasone is reported to be a potent synthetic member of the glucocorticoid class of steroid drugs. It acts as an anti-inflammatory and immunosuppressant. Glucocorticoid is reported to induce osteoporosis. On the other hand, several studies have demonstrated that dexamethasone increased the bone formation capacity of osteoprogenitor cells *in vitro*. The effects of dexamethasone on the proliferation, activity, and cytokine secretion of normal human bone marrow stromal cells were tested, and alkaline phosphatase activity was markedly stimulated with the addition

* Corresponding Author: Jun-Beom Park DDS, MSD, PhD. Department of Periodontics, Seoul St Mary's Hospital, College of Medicine, The Catholic University of Korea, 222, Banpo-daero, Seocho-gu, Seoul 137-701, Republic of Korea. Phone: +1-82-18-325-2651.

of dexamethasone. The diverse and complex effects on bone metabolism are still not completely understood.

In this paper, an extensive review of the role of dexamethasone regarding osteoblast and bone marrow stromal cells will be performed using *in vitro* and *in vivo* studies. Clinical implications of dexamethasone will be also conducted.

Keywords: Dexamethasone, osteoblast, bone, proliferation, differentiation

Introduction

Dexamethasone is a potent synthetic member of the glucocorticoid class of steroid hormones [1]. It acts as an anti-inflammatory and immunosuppressant [1]. Its potency is about 20–30 times that of hydrocortisone and 4–5 times of prednisone [1]. Dexamethasone has major effects on several organ systems, including the cardiovascular, endocrine, gastrointestinal, ophthalmic, and musculoskeletal systems [2]. Osteoporosis is reported to be one of the most serious side effects of long-term high-dose glucocorticoid therapy [3]. On the other hand, several studies have demonstrated that dexamethasone increased the bone formation capacity of osteoprogenitor cells *in vitro* [4, 5]. Its diverse and complex effects on bone metabolism are still not fully understood. The controversial effects of dexamethasone may be due to the different systems, maturation stages of the cells studied, heterogenicity of the osteoblast population, culture condition, species differences, and age of the experimental animals of used [2, 3].

In this paper, an extensive review of the role of dexamethasone regarding osteoblast and bone marrow stromal cells will be performed using *in vitro* and *in vivo* studies. Clinical implications of dexamethasone will be also conducted.

Concentration

The mean glucocorticoid (cortisone) production in man is reported to be 12.8 mg (range, 6.7-20 mg), resulting in a circulating concentration of $7x10^{-7}$M at peak levels (in the morning) and of 1×10^{-7}M at the lowest point of the circadian cycle [2]. The effects of dexamethasone may be different, depending on concentration (physiologically equivalent concentration vs. concentration at higher than physiological levels).

Proliferation

At concentration of 10^{-7}M and above, the effects on the number of cells in the primary culture of human bone marrow cells was consistently inhibitory [6]. The effects of dexamethasone on the number of human bone marrow cells were donor-dependent at concentrations of lower than 10^{-7}M [6]. The treatment of rat bone marrow stromal cells with 10^{-8}M dexamethasone increased the osteoblast cell population treated [4]. However, the treatment of human bone marrow stromal cells with dexamethasone for 24 h at a concentration of 10^{-8}M significantly suppressed [^{3}H]-thymidine incorporation, and further inhibition was observed with longer treatment [3]. Glucocorticoids at concentrations greater than 10^{-6}M inhibited osteoblast growth and proline incorporation in primary cultures of fetal rat calvaria [7, 8]. Collectively, it may be assumed that dexamethasone may increase or maintain the proliferation rate of the tested cells at a physiologically equivalent concentration, while treatment with dexamethasone may decrease the number of cells.

Osteogenic Differentiation

Human bone marrow stromal cells were examined for their osteogenic potential in an *in vitro* cell culture system [9, 10]. Dexamethasone treatment induced morphological transformation of these cells from an elongated to a more cuboidal shape and increased their alkaline phosphatase activity [9]. 10^{-8}M dexamethasone presented a significant induction in the ALP activity of human bone marrow cells [5]. Another study showed that 10^{-7}M dexamethoasone showed increased alkaline phosphatase activity, leading to osteoblast differentiation of bone marrow cells [10]. Moreover, cultures grown in the presence of 10^{-7}M dexamethasone showed higher alkaline phosphatase activity of MC3T3-E1 (osteoblast-like cell) than 10^{-8}M [11].

Inhibition of Bone Formation

Elevated levels of glucocorticoids caused by disease or therapeutic treatment of asthma and rheumatoid arthritis with glucocorticoids are known to cause bone loss, leading to osteoporosis [6, 12]. The inhibitory effect of glucocorticoids on bone formation was observed *in vivo* in animal models [13]. The glucocorticoid-induced bone loss is derived, at least in part, via inhibition of bone formation, which includes the suppression of osteoblast proliferation and collagen synthesis [3].

Mechanism

(1) Osteocalcin

The maximal stimulation of osteocalcin synthesis of rat calvarial osteoblast-like cells was also enhanced by pretreatment with 1.3×10^{-8}M dexamethasone [14].

(2) 1,25-dihydroxyvitamin D3 Receptor

Glucocorticoids are shown to increase the level of 1,25-dihydroxyvitamin D3 receptors in primary cultures of rat calvarial osteoblast-like cells [14]. Pretreatment of the cells with 1.3×10^{-8}M dexamethasone for 24 h doubled the 1,25-dihydroxyvitamin D3 receptor level without changing receptor affinity for 1,25-dihydroxyvitamin D3 and stimulated 1,25-dihydroxyvitamin D3 bioresponses.

(3) Sodium-dependent Vitamin C Transporter

Dexamethasone stimulated the update of ascorbic acid into the mouse osteoblastic cell line, specifically the MC3T3-E1 cells [15]. It was suggested that the hormone-regulated changes of the sodium-dependent vitamin C transporter expression may have an important role in cell functions including osteoblastic diffrentation.

(4) Interleukin-6 and Interleukin-11

Dexamethasone suppressed the basal inteleukin-6 and 11 secretion by human bone marrow stromal cell in a dose-dependent manner [3]. The inhibition of interleukin-6 was apparent at 10^{-9}M dexamethasone and increased with greater concentration. Dexamethasone suppressed the basal interleukin-11 at 10^{-8}M or greater concentrations.

(5) Insulin-like Growth Factor-I

Dexamethasone is reported to cause a dose-dependent inhibition of the insulin-like growth factor-I. At 10^{-8}M, dexamethasone reduced the insulin-like growth factor-I level to 70% of the control value, and at 10^{-7}M dexamethasone, the insulin-like growth factor-I level was further reduced to 60% of the control [16].

Combined Effects

(1) Calcitriol, the Active Form of Vitamin D

In rat bone marrow, adipocyte proliferation and differentiation are stimulated by glucocorticoids and calcitriol, which both act synergically, whereas osteoblastic cell proliferation and differentiation are increased by 10^{-8}M dexamethasone and inhibited by 10^{-8}M calcitriol [4].

(2) Cyclic Mechanical Strain

Levels of alkaline phosphatase were significantly increased in the dexamethasone treated group, but the effect of stretching was significantly stronger than that of dexamethasone [17]. It may be concluded that cyclical stretching and dexamethasone both enhance the osteogenic commitment of human bone marrow stromal cells.

Considerations

It was reported that the short-term application of 10^{-7}M dexamethasone led to a dose-dependent increase of cellular differentiation. Long-term use of dexamthasone seemed to reduce mineralization [11]. Similar results were achieved, such that when the chick embryo calvariae were exposed to dexamethasone from the onset of the culture, dexamethasone increased the alkaline phosphatase activity; however, when dexamethasone was added in the culture period after the bone had formed, the alkaline phosphatase activity decreased [2, 18]. It may be assumed that the effects of dexamethasone are dependent on the timing of treatment and the stage of differentiation of the osteoblast-like cells used [2].

Conclusion

A number of studies have demonstrated the effects of dexamethasone on osteogenic differentiation. Although relatively abundant information about dexamethasone indicates their possible beneficial effects on bone, there have been major side effects of long-term use of high doses of dexamethasone, including osteoporosis and leading pathologic fractures. Although dexamethasone may stimulate the differentiation of osteoprecursor cells to osteoblasts, depending on the concentration, the inhibition of proliferation in high dosages may diminish the supply of the cells and decrease bone formation.

References

[1] P. N. Naik, S. A. Chimatadar and S. T. Nandibewoor, *J. Photochem. Photobiol. B*. 100, 147 (2010).
[2] Y. Ishida and J. N. Heersche, *J. Bone Miner. Res*. 13, 1822 (1998).
[3] C. H. Kim, S. L. Cheng and G. S. Kim, *J. Endocrinol*. 162, 371 (1999).
[4] H. Atmani, D. Chappard and M. F. Basle, *J. Cell Biochem*. 89, 364 (2003).
[5] M. J. Coelho and M. H. Fernandes, *Biomaterials*. 21, 1095 (2000).
[6] S. Walsh, G. R. Jordan, C. Jefferiss, K. Stewart and J. N. Beresford, *Rheumatology (Oxford)*. 40, 74 (2001).
[7] T. L. Chen and D. Feldman, *J. Clin. Invest*. 63, 750 (1979).
[8] J. W. Dietrich, E. M. Canalis, D. M. Maina and L. G. Raisz, *Endocrinology*. 104, 715 (1979).
[9] S. L. Cheng, J. W. Yang, L. Rifas, S. F. Zhang and L. V. Avioli, *Endocrinology*. 134, 277 (1994).

[10] M. M. Beloti and A. L. Rosa, *Braz. Dent. J.* 16, 156 (2005).
[11] J. B. Park, *J. Surg. Res.* 173, 99 (2012).
[12] M. Hughes-Fulford, R. Appel, M. Kumegawa and J. Schmidt, *Exp. Cell Res.* 203, 150 (1992).
[13] A. Hulth and S. Olerud, *Br. J. Exp. Pathol.* 44, 491 (1963).
[14] T. L. Chen, P. V. Hauschka and D. Feldman, *Endocrinology.* 118, 1119 (1986).
[15] I. Fujita, J. Hirano, N. Itoh, T. Nakanishi and K. Tanaka, *Br. J. Nutr.* 86, 145 (2001).
[16] T. L. Chen, J. B. Mallory and R. L. Hintz, *Calcif. Tissue Int.* 48, 278 (1991).
[17] M. Jagodzinski, M. Drescher, J. Zeichen, et al., *Eur. Cell Mater.* 7, 35 (2004).
[18] H. C. Tenenbaum and J. N. Heersche, *Endocrinology.* 117, 2211 (1985).

Index

A

C

D

E

F

I

J

K

L

M

N

O

P

Q

R

T